many thanks for
your loving concern –
all the best,
Kerry Crofton

The Mom's Choice Awards® has recognized this book with Gold – its highest award.

Wireless Radiation Rescue – 2012

How To Use Cell Phones More Safely
and Other Safer-Tech Solutions™

Revised & Updated

Kerry Crofton, PhD

May this book bring benefit to you, your loved ones and community.

Website: www.radiationrescue.org

Published by Global WellBeing Books
First published as *Radiation Rescue* in 2009
Published as *Wireless Radiation Rescue* in 2010
This Revised & Updated Edition was published in 2012

Printed in the United States of America

Library of Congress Cataloging-in-Publication Data

Crofton, Kerry

Wireless Radiation Rescue – 2012, How To Use Cell Phones More Safely and Other Safer-Tech Solutions™ Revised & Updated

Includes resources and index.

ISBN 978-0986473531

1. Technology – health and safety. 2. Electro-magnetic radiation – Biological effects. 3. Cell phones and cancer risks. 4. Electro-pollution 5. Wireless networks and cell towers – health hazards. I. Title.

Library of Congress Control Number: 2011942182

2012 note from the author – our concern is not just cell phones

WE HUMANS, EACH WONDROUSLY UNIQUE and complex, have an inborn healthiness that is based on all the electrical fields – *within and around us* – being in harmony.

Our heart and brain cells have their own delicate electrical integrity. Our modus operandi, so to speak, relies on being attuned in this way.

We are overwhelming this natural state of wellbeing with the smog of electro-pollution, including the pulsed digital waves of radiation – from cell phones and other sources – powerful enough to blast wireless communication data through concrete. Imagine how easily this radiation travels through us, and through vulnerable children.

This book reveals why government-approved radiation emission levels from cell/mobile phones, and even baby monitors, can be harmful. Our medical team cautions us about a range of potential side effects: exposure without symptoms (harm can still be occurring), mild to moderate symptoms, electro-sensitivity, and other conditions. And, it's not only human health at risk. The good news: this is a wake-up call with easy-to-implement solutions, and pro-active strategies.

I sincerely hope that you will hear what our team of experts has to offer: how to recognize related symptoms, prevent more from developing, and how to age well with our finely-tuned, electrically-sensitive systems. We *can* reduce risks for ourselves, our children, and grandchildren. Not just ours – everyone's. We're here to help you.

Gratitude

In her 1962 ground-breaking exposé, *Silent Spring*, Rachel Carson cautioned, "Technology is often so fundamentally at odds with nature that it must be carefully monitored."

I salute the courage of Rachel Carson and the legions of other forward-thinking researchers and advocates who have endured so many battles. My gratitude also goes to those who offered us their expertise, and to the stellar team of Contributing Experts.

My appreciation goes to Sherry Lepage for her editing skill and to my beloved husband and children for their support through the long years of birthing this book, and this revised edition.

Heartfelt appreciation goes to all the people who have heard this call to protect themselves, their loved ones and their communities.

My gratitude also goes to the independent-minded media willing to hear this wake-up call. An interviewer asked me, "Don't you think the train has already left the station?" I replied, "Yes, and it's a wireless radiation hot spot. However, we can turn this around."

As you read through this book, you will see how. And why.

Quick Read at a Glance

To see if your symptoms are related to electro-pollution, check out the new 4-Day Radiation Rescue on page 49.

The section on the safer use of cell phones and headsets is from page 135 to 153, and elsewhere in the book.

Challenging the Wi-Fi in your child's school, or the cell tower in your neighborhood? See the Statement of Accountability (page 330) and the Index for research.

There's useful information in Resources on page 347.

If you want help with any health concerns: sleep problems, electro-sensitivity, or the latest anti-aging discoveries and recommendations, search our Index that begins on page 367 and at our website.

The e-Book, in all formats, is also available at our website:

www.radiationrescue.org

Contents

About the Author

Kerry Crofton is a health educator, concerned parent and member of the International EMF Alliance. She is Co-founder and Executive Director of the International Advisory Board Doctors for Safer Schools. Kerry is also Medical Commentator on electro-magnetic radiation for the American Academy of Anti-Aging Medicine's World Health Net Forum. She holds a doctorate in psychology, and her thirty-five years of professional work includes: a clinical practice; writing a weekly newspaper column on wellness issues; developing and delivering wellness programs; co-producing a television program on heart health; and directing a biofeedback clinic and hospital-based cardiac programs. Her first book, *The Healthy Type A* (Macmillan 1998), was based on these educational programs which she taught through the American and Canadian Heart Foundations. For many years, Kerry worked in the aviation industry – with pilots and air traffic controllers – and served on a judicial board, the Canadian Aviation Tribunal, enforcing the national aeronautics act.

For the past several years, Kerry has focused on electro-pollution. In researching this book, and working with prominent experts, she has become well versed in this issue. She is not a scientist; her expertise lies in health education, coaching people and organizations in effective change, and defending the public's right to know. Her clinical background has turned out to be an asset; many people dealing with electro-sensitivity, as well as digital addiction and detox, have benefitted from her counselling. Kerry has brought together the research and recommendations of leading authorities, and with their collaboration she has developed an effective plan – the basis of this book.

Introduction

Here is a brief summary for your consideration:

• increasingly powerful electronics, and other radiation exposures, are not properly tested for health safety, and the accumulated doses are not being considered – or even monitored – as far as I know;

• government standards are not accurate, and not protecting us;

• there *is* evidence of health risks, especially to our children;

• there are safer alternatives – affordable options.

You will find this book useful if:

• you have heard about cell phone radiation health hazards and want an accurate summary of the research and recommendations;

• you are ready to take action but need evidence for the doubters;

• you spend a lot of time on a computer, in a wireless environment, on a mobile phone;

• young people you care about use cell phones (mostly texting?) and you want to know which electronic devices are the safest;

• you travel in high-exposure environments like aircraft and sleep in hotels with strong Wi-Fi;

• you are concerned about the radiation from cell tower antennas, or power lines, near your home, workplace, or your children's school (and the school's wireless Internet);

• you know that you are electro-sensitive and want the best medical and technical advice for this often misdiagnosed condition;

• there's a newborn, or one about to be born, in your family and you want to know about baby monitors and other potential hazards;

And you will find this book useful if:

- you want the facts on ultrasound, airport security scanners, CT scans, MRI, X-rays and other diagnostic imaging;

- you are suffering from any of the following conditions:

  - allergies
  - ALS
  - Alzheimer's
  - ADD/ADHD
  - Asperger's Syndrome
  - Autism Spectrum Disorder
  - cancer
  - cardiac conditions - angina, arrhythmia, hypertension, tachycardia
  - cataracts
  - Chronic Fatigue Syndrome
  - depression

  - dizziness/vertigo
  - electro-sensitivity
  - epilepsy
  - headaches and migraine
  - infertility
  - insomnia
  - immune suppression
  - Multiple Chemical Sensitivity
  - tinnitus
  - Parkinson's
  - skin rashes
  - sleep disorders

- you are concerned about aging well. The effects of electro-pollution have been called "rapid aging syndrome", even aging our skin! And there's medical information on how to boost your immune system, and other longevity tips for healthy aging in this new digital age;

- a healthy balance to your family's need for electronics and screen-free time is a priority. Read about families who are unplugging and being together, outside in nature. Like you used to enjoy?

- you are interested in practical ways to protect our planet, and all life forms, from the environmental impact of electro-pollution.

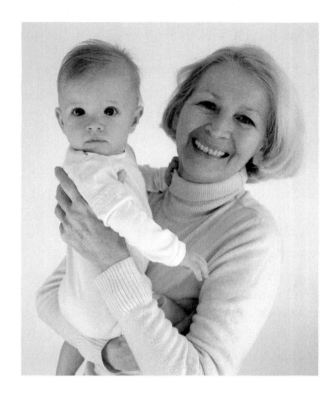

The 4 Strategies – Overview of the Book

Need to Review the Evidence?   Read through Strategy 1

If you are already well versed in the evidence, the scientists' concerns, the problem with government standards, and the misinformation, you could jump ahead to the second strategy – after you check out our new 4-Day trial on page 49. It will help you recognize and reduce sources of electro-pollution.

However, I encourage you to come back some time to the first strategy so you'll be better equipped to protect your family and educate others. If you find yourself becoming overwhelmed in Strategy 1, please skip ahead to assess your risk (Strategy 2) or to the devices and solutions section (Strategy 3), rather than abandoning this altogether.

Need to Rate Your Risks?   Strategy 2 is on page 96

Here you find a detailed questionnaire to help you see where you're being exposed to electro-magnetic fields (EMF). Some people refer to this as electro-magnetic radiation, or EMR; this is the term we'll use. We include, in simple terms, what you need to know about EMR — wired and wireless.

Need Safer Solutions?   Strategy 3 is on page 118

This offers information on everything from the lowest radiation dental X-rays, to what you need to know about tucking your child into the back seat of a hybrid car.

Details here include the kinds of cell phone headsets to avoid — and the one that is recommended, the safer alternative to cordless phones, what kind of cell phone to buy — and the best way to use it. There's also key information about safer Internet access. You'll discover practical advice about many other devices, and ways to reduce your radiation exposure and related health risks.

Need Your Action Plan?   Strategy 4 is on page 222

Here's how to create a safer environment for you and your family, room by room. Our contributing physicians also offer what you need to know about electro-sensitivity, autism, immune health, dental health and other key factors in your family's wellbeing. They also offer advice on preventing or healing from EMR exposure, and reveal how they protect their own families.

An author on parent-teen communication gives us tips on how to get young people onboard. We look at the Safer-Tech Family Challenge — this is for families wired on wireless, who take on reconnecting with each other, and the natural world around us.

Need Hope For the Future?   It is on page 326

The conclusion brings it all together with inspiration from the families following these guidelines, and from dedicated people making a difference. We hear about hopes for the future – a challenge for some who have been lone voices with their research and warnings ignored.

Resources are on page 347, and the **Index** is on page 367

There is more information at: www.radiationrescue.org

You Are The Judge and Jury In This Case

The radiation levels from devices that send and receive have been called "low" but there is enough evidence to cause concern. I am not asking you to jump to this view, but to hear the case and decide for yourself.

You can't see this kind of pollution. However, if the arcs of radiation were visible, you would see the hot zone extends a long way.

These invisible plumes of radiation surround microwave ovens, cell tower antennas, mobile phones, iPads and all wirelessly-connected devices, including video games, cordless phones and baby monitors.

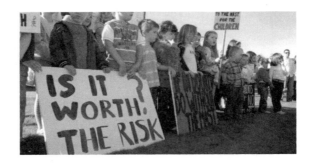

Views For You To Consider

Technical expert Grahame Blackwell, PhD, Chartered Engineer and advisor to WiredChild, explains:

> Your body is more sensitive than any wireless device, so if your device can pick up a signal, it means that your body, and your brain cells are also receiving those waves. Unlike natural sources, or radio or TV waves, the harmful frequencies from all digital devices are pulsed and jagged – like a saw tooth.

Physicians Offer Their Opinions

Many years ago, the surgeon Robert Becker, MD told us:

> Our bodies and brains generate electro-magnetic fields. We live in the Earth's natural magnetic field, and from the beginning we have been dependent on this environment.
>
> However, we have now created a vast global network of man-made electro-magnetic fields – the greatest polluting element in the earth's environment. The human body electric and the Earth's body electric have been damaged.

And in 2012 Stephen Sinatra, MD expressed concern:

> We have seen clinical evidence that electro-pollution
> affects the normal functioning of the electrically sensitive
> heart, including the rate and rhythm, and other systems
> of the body. All forms of pollution impair our health,
> and the electro-pollution arising from the proliferation
> of wireless technology has greatly added to this burden.
> The effects can go unnoticed among even the best health
> professionals. We need to educate them.

Public health expert, David Carpenter, MD, head of the Institute for
Health and Environment at the University of Albany, reported in 2011:

> There's enough science to suggest that cell phone radia-
> tion can cause cancer, but not enough political will to
> implement measures to reduce exposure. We're setting
> ourselves up for an epidemic of cancers in the future that
> should be preventable based on the knowledge we have
> now. If you use a cell phone and hold it to your head, the
> cancers you see elevated are brain cancer, tumors of the
> auditory nerve, tumors of the parotid gland, the salivary
> gland and the cheek right by the ear.

Dr. Carpenter also said that the concern is not only about cell phones.
He says there is growing evidence that people who live close to radio
towers, for example, are at increased risk of cancer:

> If your whole body is exposed, as is the case in people
> living near towers — there are studies with radio towers
> in Rome or in Korea — then the cancer that one sees
> most prominently is leukemia.

Dr. Andrew Weil, Founder and Director of the Arizona Center for Integrative Medicine, offered us this perspective:

> It's vital to focus closely on the most recently published studies, the ones that show the effects of longer-term exposure. The Environmental Working Group (EWG), a Washington, D.C.-based nonprofit organization, reported on key studies that link radiation from long-term cell phone use with increased risks of brain and salivary gland tumors, migraines and vertigo, as well as behavior problems in children, including hyperactivity.

There are many physicians opposing these views. A government health official I know, a physician with many years of medical practice, states firmly, "There is no evidence of harm from wireless technology."

Scientists State Their Findings

Dr. Devra Davis, Nobel co-laureate and a leading scientist in this field, was involved in other public health issues like tobacco. Dr. Davis tells us, "If the cell phone were a drug, it would be banned. And there's concern about other wireless devices including iPads which are even worse in terms of how much microwave radiation they emit. I am especially concerned about children and teens using mobile devices."

Professor Olle Johansson of the Karolinska Institute in Stockholm:

> There is clear evidence of harm. I am particularly concerned about children and pregnant women, and teens using mobile phones. Existing safety standards are inadequate and do not consider prolonged exposure.

Eminent scientists, including Professor Johansson, issued The Seletun Scientific Statement (*Reviews on Environmental Health* (2010; 25: 307-317) stating there is enough evidence to warrant a new approach to public health with strong preventative actions, especially concerning the growth and development of the fetus and children. They called for biologically-based exposure standards.

The World Health Organization

The 2011 report changed their long-held "no adverse effects" position on wireless radiation to "possibly carcinogenic," categorizing it with DDT, lead, engine exhaust and chloroform. The industry tried to assure us, "this doesn't mean cell phones cause cancer."

Please note: the WHO caution is *not only about cell phones* – it's about wireless microwave radiation, which would include Smart Meters, Wi-Fi, antennas/masts and other exposures. Is your child's school Wi-Fi – still using SmartBoards, iPads or wirelessly-connected computers?

The Industry Position

> Numerous scientific studies prove wireless technology is safe. This is supported by many health agencies and government standards.

What Is Your View?

This is most important as you are making the critical choices for your loved ones. This book has the research and recommendations that should be helpful for you. First, may I tell you my story? It's a journey.

We don't feel this radiation and we think it's not doing anything, but it's a very potent biological agent.

Martin Blank, PhD, Columbia University

My Wireless Wake-up Call and the 2012 Update

Oh no, you may be thinking, not another dire health warning. Like most people, I often feel fed up with alarming medical news and conflicting studies (one report implicated wine as a risk for breast cancer, and the next day another praised wine as protection from Alzheimer's Disease). What a choice!

Do you remember when it was a pleasure to sit back and read the newspaper – perhaps with a glass of wine? Most have had enough of the 'sky-is-falling' alarms. Yes, it's tempting to hang up on this wake-up call.

But please don't! There are effective solutions in this book.

First, we need to look at how we have become cocooned in convenience, in radiation hot spots, as it turns out. Realizing this hit me hard. I have been a health educator for thirty-five years yet have never faced an issue as challenging, and personally unsettling, as this one.

Briefly, here's the problem, as I understand it

As the physicians Dr. Robert Becker and Dr. Stephen Sinatra reminded us, we humans are magnificently designed bundles of energy living within the Earth's varied electro-magnetic fields.

The strong forces of the Earth, Sun and Moon affect us, and we have adapted to these. Yes, we can be killed by a bolt of lightning, or develop cancer from too much sun, but overall we have evolved to deal with this natural radiation. However, we're now in a massive soup of human-made radiation, on top of limitless numbers of new chemical toxins.

All the parents I know are concerned about raising children in an environment awash in chemical hazards. We were justly horrified to discover there was lead in toys and baby bibs, toxic Bisphenol A in plastic baby bottles, carcinogens in baby bath products, an array of chemicals in plastics, in just about everything from plastic wrap to shower curtains, and melamine in many pet foods, chocolate bars – and baby formulas!

We hear there can be traces of mercury in high fructose corn syrup, in many processed foods and sugary drinks. Mercury, one of the deadliest heavy metals, is often found in tuna from polluted oceans, in most vaccines, and 'silver' dental fillings. My dentist remarked, "If mercury is such a hazardous material it requires a strict protocol for handling, then how could your patient's mouth be a safe place to put it?" Mercury in dental fillings has been banned in Sweden and Norway.

There's also a seemingly endless list of carcinogens added to color, flavor and preserve our food; toxic chemicals added to our cosmetics, sunscreens, cleaning products, detergents and dryer sheets. Purify and freshen the air with chemically-scented candles, and plug-in, or spray, room deodorizers? What are we thinking?

Whether we're buying laundry soap, children's toys, or cell phones, are we assuming that public officials and manufacturers ensure products are rigorously tested for health effects before market? I see now that I was relying on the fox for the safety of the hen house. I hadn't realized that it evidently takes government regulators a few decades *after* a marketplace exposure before issuing public health alerts.

Remember asbestos? Tobacco? Lead? (And then, there's the story that the ancient Romans did themselves in with lead-lined wine flasks.) As you know, environmentalists have, for decades, been raising the alarm. Rachel Carson took on the chemical companies about DDT and other poisonous pesticides – and won. Carson, the mother of the environmental movement, warned us that the chemicals in our water, soil and air burden our systems and can lead to illness.

Toxic sludge and smog are, at least, hazards we can usually see. Imagine how horrified Rachel Carson would be about the environmental impact of electro-pollution, and its connection to the disappearance of the bees. And the birds. Her prediction of a silent spring now seems even more chilling. Yet I am still hopeful that people like you will listen.

As I look at the changing landscape in 2012, I am heartened by medical researchers like Dr. Carpenter speaking out. He says that the growing mass of evidence that radio-frequency fields (wireless radiation) expose people to increased risk of cancer, explains why the World Health Organization identified cell phones and radio towers as class 2B carcinogens.

That's a classification that means the evidence isn't all ~~2B~~ there but there's <u>reason to be concerned</u>. There have been several other very major advances recently — the study that came from the National Institutes of Health demonstrating directly that an active cell phone held to the head resulted in <u>changes in glucose utilization in the brain.</u> So yes, the evidence is getting strong with time.

Even though many officials still hold onto the "no evidence of harm" position, the May, 2011 WHO report is significant. Medscape Medical News reported that the WHO announcement was based on,

> ... an extensive review of studies on cell phone safety by a working group of 31 scientists from 14 countries, who met regularly to evaluate the potential carcinogenic hazards from exposure to radio-frequency fields. They reviewed exposure data, studies of cancer in humans and experimental animal models, and other relevant data.

In October, 2011 the British Medical Journal published a Danish study negating a connection between cell phones and cancer – to much media buzz. This is what many want to believe, so another "all clear" rests well. However, Dr. Davis points out that this is *not* a new study, but an extension of the 2009 study from the same Danish team – widely repudiated and not considered reliable by the WHO when they did their review. Will we hear this scientist's assessment in the news?

After the WHO report, the industry ramped up its PR campaign, as expected. There was a conference in Brussels in November, 2011 and reportedly most, if not all, of the <u>speakers were directly or indirectly linked to the telecom industry.</u> None of the scientists reporting adverse health effects, including our Contributors, were invited. This is why many people speak out strongly against industry tactics.

In the future, many consumers will wonder why they adhered to the industry's biased views and their spin on the science, and why government complacency was allowed to go on for so long. They may understand why independent scientists, including Dr. Davis, and many advocates, worked so hard to jolt people from their Wi-Fi cocoons.

And, as we've said, it isn't just human health at risk. Our authorities explain how the birds, bees and other life forms, are being adversely affected. Some of this may surprise you. Haven't we had radio and TV waves swirling around our heads, and microwave ovens and portable phones for decades? And aren't we living quite happily with wireless technology without any apparent harm?

Not even the mainstream medical community seems aware of this issue; few recognize related symptoms, conditions and risks. It has taken time, and a lot of research, to discover how to reduce our exposure without unplugging from the power grid and moving to a cabin in the woods. I'll admit, I was resistant to hearing the disturbing evidence and the onslaught of information. I didn't want this bad news.

Have you heard this: Well, everything gives you cancer, so what's the point of worrying? There's nothing we can do so why bother? Feeling overwhelmed and powerless are obstacles that can be overcome. I am hopeful that as this message is being broadcast more clearly, more people will hear not only that there is a problem, but most importantly, that there are solutions. Please remember throughout this book – and when trying to alert others – that we are, at this time, dealing with some areas of scientific uncertainty.

Yes, there is some urgency to this message.

One pioneering researcher told me, "By the time we have scientific consensus, if we ever do, we are going to have lost a lot of people."

Not my children, I protested. Now I am also fighting for yours.

I am often asked how I became so fired up about this issue – my children's wellbeing. In the spring of 2006, I was concerned about the proximity of high voltage power lines – a health hazard I knew about – too close to a new addition at our youngest child's school. Then I discovered the school's wireless Internet, and the cell tower nearby, were also putting the children at risk. Soon I was alarmed by the massive amount of eye-opening research about these health hazards.

Investigating further, I found out that many things in our environment were adding to the problem. Like most people, I carried a cell phone. I seldom used it though – instinctively it seemed that anything that could push a powerful signal through cement might not be good to press against my head. Or my children's. (You may rethink whether arming your children or teens with cell phones is really keeping them safe?) My office contained the usual must-have electronic gadgets: the latest cordless phones, a computer with wireless Internet. So convenient. Being an early adopter I brought the newest conveniences on board. And I took pride in our eco-green home. Then I had a professional electro-magnetic radiation assessment done.

Talk about an electric shock! Our youngest child's canopy bed – so beautifully decorated in pale peach and cream, with luminous stars sprinkled on the blue sky ceiling – was a hazardous hot-spot because of the radiation-reflecting metal frame. I gasped when the radiation detector screamed an alert. Who knew? I whipped that metal frame out of there before we moved on to the next room. I couldn't even bring myself to give it to anyone and thrust it into the recycling bin.

I was also shocked when the cordless portable phone sent the detector off the scale. Doesn't everyone have a cordless phone? Haven't we lived happily with this convenience for years?

The UK physician, Dr. David Dowson, urged caution, "Having a cordless phone is like having a mobile mast (a cell tower antenna) in your house." I have since replaced all our cordless phones with safer corded landlines – more details on this in Strategy 3.

Testing a friend's microwave oven was a jolt! Backing up from it, to see how far the radiation extended, I crossed her kitchen floor and almost fell down the stairs. The detector was still blaring at 25 feet (nearly 8 meters). She had known that experts say microwaves can carry health risks, so she always stood back when it was on – but not 25 feet away!

Being green at heart we had been replacing light bulbs with compact fluorescents. Guess what? Yes, they are energy-efficient but emit 'dirty electricity' (and then there's the mercury!) My husband protested, "Do you know how much energy they save?" I decided to wait to give him the news about the electric hybrid car. (You got it: sitting so close to the powerful unshielded electric battery.)

Then I learned how the radiation from the wireless router I had installed, so we could conveniently access the Internet all over the house, was also a major problem. I had no idea. As a mother, of course I am used to feeling guilty, but I truly shuddered when I realized how I had unknowingly put all of us in harm's way.

Quite honestly, I found it a lot to take in, so I understand if you are feeling overwhelmed. Like me, you may go through flashes (just what some of us don't need – more hot flashes!) of disbelief, outrage or guilt. However, I did go from being duped to determined and resolved to use my skills as a health educator to alert others. I have been working steadily ever since; sometimes inspired; often discouraged at people's unwillingness to look at this. My heart breaks when I see a pregnant woman, or a young child or teen, clutching a Blackberry, iPhone, or iPad. My frustration rises when a school insists on its Wi-Fi.

Our never-give-up team addresses a wide range of issues: from anti-aging strategies, how our children can become physiologically addicted to gaming, to the emerging concerns about wireless radiation in aircraft.

"Customers are hounding us for in-flight Wi-Fi access," an airline executive told me. If only those travellers (and pilots) knew that one of our medical contributors, Dr. Hans Scheiner, cautioned the aviation industry, "Some symptoms caused by electro-magnetic radiation like headaches, drowsiness, vertigo, nausea, loss of hearing and vision, and a lack of concentration are a concern in transportation safety, including aviation." And there can be problematic cardiac effects, as Dr. Sinatra explains. This is another reason to take this issue seriously.

Drs. Scheiner and Sinatra, and more than two dozen other authorities, have contributed to this 4-strategy plan to transform your environment into a health-enhancing, safer-tech zone, while keeping the convenience which electronics can provide.

Frequently I call upon our team to keep us up to date. For example, one of our top technical experts, Katharina Gustavs, told me of safer baby monitors available in Europe. Why wouldn't we choose this option?

I speak to you as a mother and a health educator. Working together, we *can* meet this challenge. You have my personal commitment to help you, your family, and your community as much as I can.

It's Your Decisions That Matter

Remember, our goal is for you to have the information you need to safeguard your loved ones, maintain your health, and age well in this wireless world.

Now, please allow me to introduce our dedicated team.

Contributing Researchers, Clinicians and Technical Experts

Martin Blank, PhD – Associate Professor of Physiology and Cellular Biophysics at Columbia University;

Carolyn Dean, MD, ND – physician and naturopathic doctor specializing in complementary medicine and environmental health;

Professor Devra Davis, PhD – founder of Environmental Health Trust, Nobel Co-laureate and award-winning epidemiologist;

Leslie S. Feinberg, DC – chiropractor and developer of the energy medicine treatment NeuroModulation Technique;

Larry Gust – electrical engineer and Institute for Bau-Biologie® (IBE) certified Building Biologist;

Katharina Gustavs – Building Biology environmental consultant specializing in electro-magnetic field testing and environmental and occupational health;

Stan Hartman – environmental health consultant with Radsafe in Boulder, CO specializing in EMF/EMR issues;

Magda Havas, PhD – Associate Professor of Environmental and Resource Studies at Trent University;

Carrie Hyman, LAc, OMD – licensed acupuncturist and Doctor of Chinese Medicine who was an associate professor at the California Acupuncture College;

Olle Johansson, PhD – Associate Professor at the Department of Neuroscience, Karolinska Institute and Professor at The Royal Institute of Technology, Stockholm, Sweden;

Vini Khurana, MD – Neurosurgeon at the Canberra Hospital, and Associate Professor of Neurosurgery at Australian National University Medical School;

Dietrich Klinghardt, MD, PhD – physician practicing in the US and Europe and founder of the Klinghardt Academy of Neurobiology which offers in-depth training programs for health practitioners;

Henry Lai, PhD – Research Professor, Department of Bio-engineering, School of Medicine and College of Engineering, University of Washington;

Heather McKinney, PhD – researcher who specializes in strategic planning for effective change and health improvement within individuals, organizations and communities;

Rob Metzinger – Electronics Engineering Technologist, and instructor and consultant with the International Institute for Bau-Biologie® (IBE);

Alasdair Philips – the Director of Powerwatch (UK), qualified in Electrical and Electronic Engineering;

William Rea, MD – former surgeon who founded the Environmental Health Center in Dallas, Texas and one of the world's leaders in environmental medicine;

Hans Scheiner, MD – physician practicing complementary medicine in Germany, has treated thousands of electro-sensitive patients in his medical clinic;

Peter Sierck – industrial hygienist with IBE and IBN certification who has more than twenty years of experience performing professional EMF and RF measurements;

Stephen Sinatra, MD, FACC, CNS – board-certified cardiologist, Fellow in the American College of Cardiology, founder of Heart MD Institute, and writes a newsletter entitled *Heart, Health & Nutrition*;

Louis Slesin, PhD – founder and publisher of Microwave News, the newsletter which was established in 1980 and is now online;

Sarah Starkey, PhD – neuroscientist in the UK with a specific concern about wireless systems in the school environment;

Jacob Teitelbaum, MD – author of *From Fatigued to Fantastic* and a specialist in complementary medicine.

All of us can benefit from the dedication of our contributing experts.

May I also recommend these excellent documentaries.

Full Signal

Several of our experts appear in the 2010 award-winning film *Full Signal*, by the veteran journalist and director Talal Jabari. This compelling 61-minute film features scientists, activists, lawyers and lawmakers. It is an excellent way to communicate this message to your community, or school board – available at www.fullsignalmovie.com.

Disconnect: A Film About Cell phones & Radiation

This 2011 documentary is by filmmaker Kevin Kunze. Through research and interviews with Dr. Devra Davis, author of the book *Disconnect: The Truth About Cell phone Radiation* (Plume, 2011) and other leading scientists, politicians, activists and victims, this film traces the rise of a rogue industry and explains why many experts believe brain tumors, infertility, and breast cancer are correlated with cell phone use. It features people who helped shape the cell phone industry including Apple's co-founder Steve Wozniak, Virgin Mobile's founder Richard Branson, and head of one of the first telecom companies – more details: www.kevinkunze.com and www.environmentalhealthtrust.org.

Protecting Our Children and Other Success Stories

Some are leading the way and replacing wireless Internet with wired

As a school principal, I see the health and safety of our children as a non-negotiable responsibility. Although there is far from universal agreement as to the dangers of wireless technology, and there are many with vested interests in its continued use, evidence of harm is extensive. The default position must be on the side of safety. I have removed all wireless technology from our school and banned the use of cell phones within our building. In our older classes, every child has a laptop, connected to the internet through a hard-wired cable. We have advanced technology without the dangers of wireless radiation.

Kristin Cassie, Principal, Roots & Wings Montessori, British Columbia

Other educators have replaced Wi-Fi including three Ontario schools: In 2010 the parents' council at St. Vincent Euphrasia Elementary in Meaford voted for a hard-wired system. In 2011, also citing health concerns, Pretty River Academy in Collingwood and Wayside Academy in Peterborough took this step. Why expose students (and staff) to a known health hazard when there are safer, and more efficient, options readily available? Are your children and grandchildren facing this risk?

2 Minute Quick Read Summary

Strategy 1. Know the Evidence

WE ARE ADAPTIVE BEINGS who have adjusted well to the other electrical fields in our environment. Until now.

Electro-magnetic radiation from massive man-made wireless and wired exposures has been shown to cause harmful effects, especially to children.

Some of the adverse biological effects:

- damage to our DNA;

- suppression of the immune system;

- leakage of the blood-brain barrier;

- thickening of the blood.

There are also other harmful effects to the cardiovascular, neurological and endocrine systems.

Why bother with yet another health concern? 30 minutes a day on your cell phone, over 10 years, can increase your risk of brain cancer by 40% (Interphone study) or as much as 140% (Professor Hardell). How many minutes a day do you spend on a cell phone, or a new high-powered multi-media device? And having wireless Internet and cordless phones in your home could be the reason you are not sleeping well.

See Strategy 1 for more details.

The voluntary exposure of the brain to microwaves from hand-held mobile phones is the largest human biological experiment ever.

Professor Salford, MD, Lund University, Sweden

Strategy 1. Know the Evidence

- the levels of electro-magnetic radiation that we are exposed to today are billions of times higher than for our ancestors (yes, *billions*, and this is a conservative estimate);

- this technology was never pre-market tested for safety;

- the current government standards we assume are protecting us are, evidently, just plain wrong;

- **fortunately, there is good news** - this is not an insurmountable problem; there are safer solutions and hope on the horizon.

Facts do not cease to exist because they are ignored. Aldous Huxley

Microwaving this Blue Planet

As if satellites hovering over us in space, city-wide canopy wireless systems, and powerful electrical grids weren't enough, Mt. Everest – "the roof of the world" – has become another radiation hot spot. And on the horizon, there's also increasingly wide-ranging "blitzkrieg" Wi-MAX networks, all-wireless homes, and even more powerful wireless devices –"Wi-Fi on steroids"– as one tech writer announced with glee. You may be wondering if many scientists report evidence of harm, then why haven't our governments done something to protect us? And, how did wireless devices make it to market in the first place?

Good questions. Let's jump in and take a quick look at that. Could your cell phone heat your coffee? If not, it was considered safe.

Why Government Regulations Are Not Protecting Us

Our safety standards were, and still are, only based on thermal damage. Thermal means that the energy has the ability to heat, and non-thermal means it does not. Way back in the techno dark ages – the early nineties – regulators only considered thermal effects. This was not the ability to *cook* tissue, just warm it.

Because short-term exposure from cell phones did *not* heat the tissue of a 200 lb adult male, the industry argued wireless devices were safe and should be excluded from pre-market testing. Potential damage to smaller, more vulnerable, beings was *not* tested, or considered. Professor Gandhi – his graphic of the skulls is on the book cover – worries about this, "All the standards used for cell phones apply only to the 'big guy' brain." How is this oversight affecting your children?

Unbelievably, this is still the only thing that government regulations are based on, and still govern the marketplace. And you should know that the standards for radiation emitted from your cell phone, wireless network, cordless phone, baby monitor, or nearby cell tower antenna are not a little bit off; they are *thousands to millions* of times apart from what many eminent scientists consider safe.

So why are our schools installing Wi-Fi? And hospitals. And parks. And planes. No government agencies seem to be monitoring the impact on human health – on us – or considering the affect in five years. In two?

Professor Johansson cautions:

> People should know about the difference between acute (immediate) and long-term health effects. The current standards only look at acute effects.

As you see, we need to take a course of action to safeguard our families, and not wait for regulators and public health officials to wake up.

Government Regulators are "just plain wrong"

The environmental health physician, Dr David Carpenter, made that hard-hitting statement. Remember this when you have concerns about the wireless at your children's school, question the cell tower antenna, or ask about cell phone safety. You may get: "The radiation levels fall well within government standards." Public health officials may insist, "There is no clear evidence of harm." The industry also holds to these positions. Here are some questions you could ask .

7 Key Questions

1. Are those standards up to date? (In the US, not since 1997, when the FCC first set exposure limits. Internationally – ICNIRP in 1998.)

2. Have these levels been proven safe for women, children, pregnant women, or the fetus? (RF exposure tests were based on short-term, thermal – heating – effects, only considering adult males.)

3. Did they investigate long-term, and/or non-thermal effects? (No, and brain cancer can take 10-30 years to develop; 3 years for leukaemia in children. While DNA damage, leakage of the blood-brain barrier, cognitive impairment, sperm damage and cardiac effects can occur within a short time at those 'low' government-approved levels.

4. Have you, as an official/expert, taken steps, like many European countries, to re-evaluate these standards, and recommend precautions?

5. Will you, as an official/expert, give us your personal assurance that the standards you are upholding are safe, and tell us if there are any published, or unpublished, exposure restrictions? We assert our right to know why you are defending this position if you refuse to sign. (See Statement of Accountability on page 330.)

6. What agency is monitoring any adverse health effects, including wireless Internet access in aircraft, or other modes of transportation?

7. What agency is measuring the cumulative dose we are being subjected to, and the potential impact, even if we don't use a cell phone, or have removed wireless exposures from our homes?

Remember the headlines "Talk all you want—it's safe!"

When I tried to tell people about this, most didn't want to believe it. People often pointed to a well-publicized, and controversial, Danish study that was released in 2006. I have learned the importance of having a critical eye when reading such research papers. In the case of that Danish study, scientists not working for the industry found serious flaws. Evidently, the trouble with many studies that show no increased risk with cell phone use is that significant information may be missing.

What is happening in Denmark? In 2009, a different Danish study reported, "No increase in brain tumors seen from cell phones" was widely repudiated by independent experts. Another Danish study in 2011 was also widely criticized. How are we, the consumers, to know?

Wait until you hear what our experts have to reveal about the Interphone study released in 2010. Independent researchers report that studies don't always ask what side of the head the person uses the phone on – a key variable in assessing risk. People are included as users even if they only had rare or occasional exposure. Also, only a very small proportion of the population had cell phones 10-15 years ago, and it can take 10 years or more for a tumor to develop. These studies wouldn't necessarily provide clear cause and effect. How many decades, and thousands of studies, did it take before it was "proven" that smoking caused cancer?

Evidence is Building

If it can take so many years to see evidence of the damage what does this mean to a whole generation using cell phones day and night? Is it prudent to wait?

Those saying there's no problem, or who do not take precautionary action – in the face of growing signs of harm – may have a lot to answer for, one doctor confided to me.

Dr. David Servan-Schreiber, Professor of Psychiatry at the University of Pittsburgh, and Dr. Annie Sasco who worked with the World Health Organization agree that there are cell phone health concerns:

> What we have now are highly suggestive results from a number of different studies…that point to a non-negligible long-term risk for a brain tumor.

Dr. Magda Havas, from the Environmental and Resource Studies Program, Trent University, confirms other risks:

> Headaches, numbness and tingling sensations in their fingers and face, and difficulty with cognitive functions either when using, or being in the presence of, cell phones and/or cordless phones. Also, people who live within 400 meters (437 yards) of the antennas are experiencing adverse health symptoms. Studies show an increase in cancers and symptoms of what is being called electro-hypersensitivity or EHS.

Biased Evidence in Industry-Funded Studies?

Dr. Henry Lai is one of a number of credible scientists who have faced attempts to discredit their findings. The trouble started when Dr. Lai's work at the University of Washington showed that radiation at frequencies similar to those emitted by cell phones broke the DNA in rats' brain cells after just two hours of exposure (Lai & Singh 2004).

In "The Cellphone Game", an excellent article published in the September 2008 edition of The Walrus magazine, Dr. Lai reports:

Industry-funded studies are roughly twice as likely as government-funded ones to conclude that cell phones are harmless.

The next time you hear about a study, or an expert of some sort, saying that cell phones are safe, may I suggest you follow the funding.

The Controversial Interphone Study

This is a good example of why many people are confused. One of the reasons I wrote this book is to help consumers, especially parents like me, sort out the science behind such headlines as "Interphone study inconclusive, cell phones safe, after all." I wish this were true.

This massive study began in the late 1990s with researchers from 13 countries investigating the possible tumor risks associated with the use of mobile phones. I asked Dr. Louis Slesin, editor of Microwave News, for his insider's perspective, as he has been following this:

> Several of the research groups, including Lennart Hardell's team, reported that there *is* statistically significant evidence of two different kinds of tumors from cell phone use of ten years, or more, on the same side of the head as the phone was used. It is baffling how some other Interphone members can be so sure that cell phones are safe. No one should forget that the wireless industry plays a huge role in this area of research.

For updates go to www.microwavenews.com – a reliable source.

The definition of a 'heavy user' has changed since Interphone began. If you have been on your cell phone only *30 minutes a day* over a 10-year period, then you'd qualify as an Interphone *'heavy user'*, with a 40 percent increased risk of a brain tumor. If you use a cell phone twice as much – *60 minutes a day,* would that mean your risk is doubled?

If it's only *4 minutes a day* (the amount the average person in this study used a cell phone) then you fall comfortably into the Interphone 'no conclusive link' category – as long as you are not exposed to other sources of wireless radiation.

How many hours a day of wireless radiation exposure is your family accumulating? Ever check your bill? You may have a great savings plan, but what about the cost to your health?

Did you know that the Interphone researchers did not consider:

- the exposure time when your cell phone is on standby, you carry it on your body, use it as an alarm, or charge it beside your bed;
- the increased risk incurred by young adults, teens, children or pregnant women;
- other exposures including cordless phones, wireless networks etc.

Worth waiting for the end of this debate before taking action?

As you know, people of all ages are fixated on their multi-media mobiles which are so convenient, and so cool, with their dazzling apps. You can chat and text, catch the news and weather, download movies and locate a restaurant. Now, from a stunning display tablet, you can also watch TV and spend hours at work or play. Note: whenever you are online, sending and receiving, this is all Wi-Fi – microwave radiation exposure.

These gadgets are powerful enough to send and receive data through your parking garage. Does it seem wise to press one, with its intense hot-spot plume, against your head? Your heart? Your unborn baby?

There are many groups joining the Interphone call for more research, including the 2010 US report from The President's Cancer Panel. Yes, independent research is of value. It seems to me, however, we already have lots of strong evidence of harm.

Let's take a look at the various systems of the body that are affected. You will see why so many symptoms and medical conditions can be related. The good news: there are many health benefits when you reduce your exposure with our safer-tech solutions.

This section gives you a detailed list of potential effects. Why are we still standing and not crashing under all this wireless radiation? A good question. Noticeable harm can be immediate, or take many years.

Biological Effects – Evidence of Damage

Yes, there *are* numerous peer-reviewed and published studies that strongly suggest harmful effects. Here we go ...

Functioning of Our Cells

Scientists now have far more sensitive measures of how human cells respond to EMR than they did in the 1990s.

As the research of Dr. Blank demonstrates, these fields can affect our cells even when present at very low intensities – low enough that our senses can't detect them, let alone feel any heat. (Could this be the crux of the problem?)

Along with Dr. Reba Goodman, Dr. Blank has been studying these biological effects on the stress response in cells. He explains for us how the cells interpret this stimulus.

> The cells react as if this energy is harmful! They make stress proteins only when they sense they're in a bad situation, such as when they are exposed to heat, toxins or the wrong pH. The research is showing that when

exposed to low frequency they're responding in this way, even without thermal stressors. When the cell starts making stress proteins, it's trying to tell you something!

There are other troubling signs of reactivity. In 2011 Drs. Blank and Goodman published a new paper on DNA in the *International Journal of Radiation Biology 87(4): 409-15, 2011.* This review of the responses of DNA to electro-magnetic fields, in different frequency ranges, shows that the DNA in cells can react as a fractal antenna, able to pick up many frequencies. This property of DNA is probably due to its structure. This DNA damage could account for increases in cancer.

Our Immune and Other Systems

Another scientist, Dr. Ted Litovitz, who was Emeritus Professor of Physics and Bioelectro-magnetics, Catholic University of America, Washington, DC, found that when a cell is subjected to too much stress, this fundamental protective response itself becomes stressed and stops making proteins. (Litovitz 2002) In other words, the cell becomes less able to protect itself and this impairs our immune system strength and affects every system in the body.

Our Cells' Ability to Communicate

The pioneer in the field of environmental health, Dr. Neil Cherry of New Zealand, described this mechanism in detail. Sadly, this highly respected scientist died in 2003 after suffering from Motor Neuron disease (ALS). Professor Cherry wrote:

> Nature has developed many advanced and complex biological processes in, and between, cells for cell-to-cell communication, intra-cellular communication and regulation, and brain and CNS systems. Dr. Ross Adey's

description of cells 'whispering to each other' in this cell-to-cell caring society, checking on the health of their neighbours and suggesting subtle changes to keep them healthy are part of biological homeostasis.

Our brains and cells primarily use calcium ions for these processes and Dr. Adey's laboratory, followed by Dr. Carl Blackman's monumental work, confirms that the natural and vital processes for cellular health are interfered with ... at the cell membrane level, by the oscillating signals from mobile phone base stations.

These waves of radiation confuse and damage the cell's signal system while the strong emissions of a cell phone next to your head almost drown out the signals. This alters the EEG and hormones, damaging the cells and producing acute symptoms such as headache, concentration problems, memory loss, dizziness and nausea, and long-term problems including brain tumors, Alzheimer's Disease, depression and suicide.

The cardiologist Dr. Stephen Sinatra told me about this hypothesis:

Receptor sites on the cell membrane do not recognize the chaotic electrical disturbances from mobile phones and other wireless exposures, and interpret this as a foreign invader, sending the cell membranes into a protective 'lock down' mode.

One theory is that electro-magnetic radiation (EMR) impedes the active transport channels that should allow nutrients into the cell, and waste products to get out, as well as the cells' ability to communicate and work well with each other. Waste products can build up inside the cell causing a high concentration of molecules called free radicals.

Our DNA

Free radicals interfere with DNA repair and alter future DNA. Damaged DNA is passed along to the next generation of cells. This is worrying, because, as Adey explains, the cells can no longer 'whisper' with each other, they can no longer call in the immune system to remove dead cells and damaged DNA.

The researchers Drs. Henry Lai and Narendra Singh have been studying DNA for many years, and their results are strong evidence. Even with brief exposures, at very low levels of EMR, there are signs of significant damage to DNA, and they report this can lead to changes in cellular functions and cell death. (This study, with J.L. Philips, was published in *Pathophysiology* 16 (2009) 79–88.) I asked Dr. Lai and Dr. Singh about security scanners and our DNA — more on that later.

This disruption to the normal functioning of cells affects all life forms, not just us wireless-crazed humans. One of Dr. Hyman's presentations is titled *The Inconvenient Truth About Convenient Technology*. She cautions:

> This radiation affects every living cell in ways we are only beginning to understand. Because of the genotoxic effect of radio frequencies in particular, we may be altering the genetic expression of all life on earth.

Our Cardiovascular System

Having worked for many years in the field of heart health education, I welcomed Dr. Sinatra's contribution and peppered him with questions about the possible connection between EMR and cardiac symptoms.

Even if you have never had any worrying cardiac symptoms, you'll find what he says of interest:

> The heart is electrical in nature so it is vulnerable to all electro-magnetic fields. These include the earth's natural forces – as strange as this may sound, ask any cardiologist who has worked in the ER on a full moon night – as well as the microwaves from wireless technologies.
>
> The non-harmonious, jagged waveform of wireless radiation impairs the normal functioning of the heart, including the rate and rhythm.
>
> Some people can feel discomfort in the chest area when around mobile phones or wireless hot spots.
>
> People are usually unaware of the cause of these 'unexplained' cardiac symptoms, and unknowingly, their doctors may not offer the appropriate diagnosis, or treatment. Even if you are not aware of any effects, it does not mean that you are safe from harm.
>
> Cardiac effects may include: variability of heart rate and rhythm (tachycardia and arrhythmia), palpitations, chest discomfort/pain (angina), high blood pressure (hypertension - this is now better understood: oxidative stress/free radical damage from toxins, environmental

pollution, emotional stress etc. impairs the delicate lining of small blood vessels, causing constriction and an increase in blood pressure), blood clumping (this thickening of the blood also happens with the stress response, as you can imagine, thicker, more viscous blood is not a healthy condition).

Our Blood-Brain Barrier

Even though this is a complex mechanism, this research caught my attention – like the graphic on the back cover. I read that the "lock down" effect of the cell membrane by EMR can affect cells anywhere in the body – including the blood-brain barrier, a vital filtering system in the blood vessels in the brain.

Experts agree that it's especially important that the cells of the blood-brain barrier keep toxins out and cerebrospinal fluids in, so that the environment of the brain is kept clean and the brain itself is cushioned against any contact with the skull. Makes sense.

Research by Leif Salford, MD, the neurology professor at Lund University, shows that EMR is capable of causing leakage of the blood-brain barrier. (Persson and Salford 1996; Salford et al. 1992, 1993, 1994, 1997b, 2001)

Strategy 1. Know the Evidence

Dr. Salford's research team reported rat brain cross-sections showed first ever evidence of brain damage from cell phone radiation. While the controls (top) appeared healthy, the test subjects (below) – exposed to a 2-hour dose of cell phone radiation of varying intensities – were heavily spotted with proteins leaked from the surrounding blood vessels, and show signs of significant neuronal (brain) damage.

I once showed this graphic to a neurologist. He looked right at me and challenged: "Do you have any idea of the implications of this kind of damage?"

"I am beginning to understand," I replied. "This is why I am so committed to getting this information out to people – particularly to parents like me."

Maybe you're thinking that what applies to rat brains doesn't necessarily apply to humans? Several years ago, Professor Salford pointed out that the blood-brain barrier is anatomically the same in both species and cautioned:

> With a long series of significant effects demonstrated in the animal models, it is my sincere belief that it is more probable than unlikely that non-thermal electro-magnetic fields from mobile phones do have effects upon the human brain.

Our Cognitive Abilities

A 2009 study by researchers in Israel confirmed human subjects exposed to wireless radiation from cell phones had impaired cognitive functions, including slower response times to a spatial working memory task (Luria, Eliyahu, Hareuveny, Margaliot, Meiran).

So why are we flooding schools with wireless radiation?

I challenged one skeptical principal with this question. If the safety of the school's playground equipment was being questioned by highly respected scientists, and there were reports of children being harmed, and at risk, how long would it take you to remove it from the school grounds? (More information on this at www.doctorsforsaferschools.org).

Neurological Conditions, Including ADHD and Autism

There are many symptoms connected with EMR exposure including difficulty sleeping, headaches, dizziness, eye pain, cardiovascular reactions, and many more. Sadly, medical researchers also suggest an extensive range of brain and nervous system-related conditions.

These include: learning disabilities, ADD and ADHD, Asperger's Syndrome and the Autism Spectrum Disorders, MS, ALS, Parkinson's and Alzheimer's Disease.

A 2003 published study by Professor Salford suggests an EMR and Alzheimer's link; with 4 billion cell phone users, if microwave radiation turns out to be a causative factor what will we do?

Some years ago, studies reported a link between electrical occupations and neuro-degenerative disease including ALS (Suavity et al, 1998). I know several people afflicted with this devastating condition, and some with Parkinson's. They were otherwise healthy men in their 50's and 60's – all worked in the computer industry. If there is a connection, what impact could this have on the digital generation? This seems worth an investigation and taking precautions.

There is also concern about the rising levels of Autism Spectrum Disorder (ASD). More and more families are facing this every day: a few decades ago autism struck 1 in 10,000 children; now it affects 1 in every 150, according to a study released in February 2007 by the CDC (Centers for Disease Control and Prevention). In October 2009, a new government study estimates that the prevalence is more likely about 1 in every 91 children. What could it be in 2019?

There is some good news; as an environmental consultant who assists families with autism tells us later on, many of these children improve significantly when in a low EMR environment. This is not the whole answer we need, but it is a fairly low-cost, and easy-to-implement, plan.

Our Memory

Yes, this critical function dims as we age, but there's an EMR factor, according to the neuroscientist Professor Olle Johansson:

If you look in the literature, you have a large number of various effects like chromosome damage, impact on the concentration capacity, and decrease in short term memory.

Memory loss and concentration problems may occur as radiation affects the ability of the brain to process and remember information (part of distracted driving?), and can damage and kill brain cells, most of which do not re-grow. This could be a factor in dementia.

Our Skin

We have just heard about free radical damage to our DNA; there's more. Dr. Benetti, at the French company, Clarins Laboratories, exposed skin cells to EMR and found it damaged the quality of the skin, accelerating the aging process by causing a production of free radicals and a loss of cellular renewal. The skin became dehydrated, more sensitive, and less radiant. They are developing plant-based protective formulas.

Our Breasts

Research indicates damage from wireless communication – time spent on cordless, or cell, phones – can include risk of breast cancer. There's evidence that breast tissue absorbs electro-magnetic radiation. Isn't that awful news. All of us have lost loved ones – wonderful women. This is a good reason to avoid carrying a powered-on cell phone on your body, and to limit its use. (I have seen mobile phones as pendants.)

All this evidence is too scary?

We may fear for ourselves, and our family. My hope is you'll see that if environmental influences are part of these diseases, then we can prevent, and treat, them, more effectively, but that long list *is* daunting. Once I submitted an article to an editor who rejected it as "too scary". We may not want to hear this, sadly, we need to. However, if you are feeling overwhelmed, maybe it's time to put down this book and go for a brisk walk in the fresh air?

Pre-natal Exposure

Here's published evidence that expectant parents, and their doctors, should read.

• <u>Birth defects</u> and proximity to high voltage power lines. Reprod Toxicol. 1993 May-Jun; 7(3) 283-7. Childhood leukemia is also linked with proximity to power lines.

• RF exposure (from wireless radiation) and adverse effects on the <u>developing fetal</u> brain. Nakamichi N, Ishioka Y, Hirai T, Ozawa S, Tachibana M, Nakamura N, Takarada T, Yoneda Y. Journal Neuroscience Research, August 2009, Volume 87, Issue 11, Pages 2399–2614

• RF exposure and possible promotion of neuronal differentiation in fetal rat brain neural progenitor cells. Nakamichi N, et al. Journal Neuroscience Research 2009, Aug 15;87(11):2406-17.

And there's new evidence from researchers presenting at the June, 2011 conference in Istanbul – on offspring subjected to EMR exposure (the babies of animals exposed to common levels of wireless radiation):

• Rabbits and rats – evidence of damage to the fetal brain, eyes, liver and skin. A. Tomruk, Gazi University, Ankara.

• Abnormal changes in different types of fetal brain cells and structure. Prof. Sulleyman Kaplan, Ondokuz Mayis University, Samsun.

• Biomarkers of genetic and other damage to fetal cells and organs. Prof. Nesrin Seyhan et al. Gazi University. None of this sounds good, does it?

How much evidence do you need to take action to protect your baby?

If pre-natal EMR exposure has the potential to damage offspring, and if nursery exposure can harm babies, could these be factors in sudden infant death syndrome?

Childhood Cancers

In Australia, the UK and Italy, studies found that the closer people live to broadcast towers (radio and/or TV transmitters) the higher their incidence of leukemia (Michelozzi 2001, 2002, Hocking et al 1996.) Other studies looked at people living near power lines – with a small increase in the number of power lines, there was a doubling of childhood leukemia by age 3 or 4 (Draper et al 2005).

For 30 years experts have investigated how EMR could increase the risk of childhood leukemia. In 2008, medical researchers in Shanghai, led by Xiaoming Shen, reported a ground-breaking theory: children who carry a defective gene that normally helps repair damaged DNA are up to 4 times more likely than neighboring children, with a fully-functioning gene, to develop leukemia, if they also live near power lines or transformers. They report that children who have this faulty gene cannot repair DNA that's damaged by EMR, even low frequency fields. This impairment could increase their risk of cancer.

A mother's exposure in her work environment during pregnancy, or just before she conceives, may also put her child at greater risk of developing certain types of brain cancer. In February 2009, researchers at Canada's McGill University raised this concern after following the pregnancies of women working on electric sewing machines. And there are new reports that pre-natal exposure to cell phone radiation may increase the risk of glioma in the offspring, and a range of electro-magnetic fields may be a factor in infertility and miscarriages.

To many EMR researchers, a pregnant woman chatting on her iPhone, or resting a Blackberry, or laptop, on her ample abdomen, appears as shocking as seeing her smoking or drinking alcohol. The new health warning during pregnancy: refrain from drugs, alcohol, tobacco, prolonged proximity to electric devices, and avoid mobile technology.

As with tobacco, and other public health issues, there's usually a long time lag between people getting sick and governments taking action, as we mentioned. Not only are the agencies in charge not stepping in to fund needed research and provide necessary precautions, most are still defending the existing 'safe' levels which respected scientists warn are not protecting us. Meanwhile, reports from the European Union alert us that childhood brain cancers are on the rise.

British neurosurgeon Kevin O'Neill, MD has reported:

> Brain tumours are on the increase, reportedly in the region of 2% per year. But in my unit we have seen **the number of cases nearly double in the last year.**

Some scientists and epidemiologists fear we may face a global pandemic of brain cancer. How much does the convenience really mean to us, when we consider such risks? We feel harrowed seeing the bright face, and shiny bald head, of one child with cancer. How would we cope with many? There are dedicated researchers and message carriers, around the world, fighting hard to prevent this. We need your help.

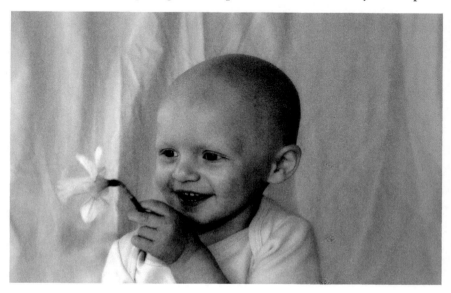

Dr. Davis is particularly concerned about our children:

> When it comes to proof of human harm, we've kind of been led down a garden path that says the only proof that really counts is enough sick or dead people. I think that approach has got to change, and particularly with respect to something like brain cancer.
>
> Brain cancer can take 10, 20 or 30 years to develop. It may affect people 30, 40 years after they've been exposed.
>
> Our children are using cell phones in growing numbers. They're marketing cell phones now to five-year-olds...
>
> Should we wait until we have proof of sick, or dead, kids before acting? I don't think so, and neither does the European parliament.

Dr. Louis Slesin is another strong voice urging more research:

> Here's the killer: there is not a single study on cell phone radiation going on in the United States today. Nothing. There's a big study in the wings, but it hasn't started yet. But if that gets under way, we'll have one study. That's it.
>
> Now, with four billion people worldwide using cell phones, could we spend a few dollars finding out whether our children are at risk or not?

A Partial Summary of EMR Biological Effects

"No evidence of harm," some claim. However, even at low

levels EMR is bio-active, every part of the body is affected and published evidence includes:

- DNA damage and disruption of DNA repair (Lai, Singh, Philips)

- Suppression of the immune system (Johansson, Nakamura, Litovitz, Veyret, Hocking, Draper)

- Disruption to normal functioning of neurological, cardiovascular and endocrine systems (Lai, Salford, Becker, Cherry, Hurtado, Johansson, Karasek, Schilowsky)

- Leakage of the brain's protective blood-brain barrier (Salford, Persson)

- Impaired cognitive functions, including reaction time (Mosgoeller, Scheiner, Lai, Becker, Cherry, Luria, Eliyahu, Hareuveny, Margaliot, Meiran)

- Increased agitation, sleep disruptions and food, chemical and electro-sensitivities (Becker, Holt, Rea)

- Stress protein synthesis (body's reaction when stressed at the cellular level) (Blank, Goodman, Mosgoeller)

- Inter- and intra-cellular functions (cell membrane permeability and the cells ability to communicate with each other) (Cherry, Adey, Blackman)

More Evidence of Harm

Building Biology consultant and Industrial Hygienist, Peter Sierck, with his colleague Thomas Haumann PhD, offer this summary of non-thermal biological effects from wireless technologies. (Nonstop Pulsed 2.4 GHz Radiation Inside US Homes) You can show this to your friend (or government agency, or industry spokesperson) who protests, 'there is no real evidence of harm'.

"Much experimental evidence of non-thermal influences of microwave radiation on living systems has been published in the scientific literature during the last 30 years – relating both to in vitro and in vivo studies.

- Changes in the electrical activity in the human brain,
- Increase in DNA single and double strand breaks from HF exposure to 2.45 GHz,
- Increased lymphoma rates (2 fold) in transgenic mice exposed twice a day to 30 minutes of cell phone (GSM) signals over 18 months,
- Increased permeability of the blood-brain barrier in rats,
- Observation of an increase in resting blood pressure during exposure,
- Increased permeability of the erythrocyte membrane,
- Effects on brain electrochemistry (calcium efflux),
- Increase of chromosome aberrations and micronuclei in human blood lymphocytes,
- Synergistic effects with cancer promoting and certain psychoactive drugs,
- Depression of chicken immune systems,
- Increase in chicken embryo mortality,
- Effects on brain dopamine/opiate electrochemistry,
- Increases in DNA single and double strand breaks in rat brain,
- Stressful effects in healthy and tumor bearing mice,
- Neurogenetic effects and micronuclei formation in peritoneal macrophage."

Brain Cancer and More Medical Warnings

As I mentioned, no one seems to be measuring, or monitoring, the combined daily dose of radiation we receive from wired and wireless exposures. Even if we don't use a cell phone; we are not escaping.

David Carpenter, MD, Director, Institute for Health and the Environment at the University of Albany and co-author of The BioInitiative Report warns:

> **This report stands as a wake-up call that long-term exposure to some kinds of EMF may cause serious health effects.**
>
> Good public health planning is needed now to prevent cancers and neurological diseases linked to exposure to power lines and other sources of EMF. We need to educate people and our decision-makers that 'business as usual' is unacceptable.

It is still an uphill battle, as you can imagine. In 2008 Dr. Carpenter testified at a US Congressional hearing along with Dr. Ronald B. Herberman, an internationally recognized tumor immunologist. They stated that according to the government's own statistics, the incidence of brain cancer has been increasing over the last ten years, particularly among 20-29 year-olds.

If it takes more than ten years for brain tumors to grow, and if these are, in fact, being caused by cell phones, cancer rates might not peak for at least another five years, in Dr. Herberman's opinion. Then what?

You see why I jumped in to safeguard my family without waiting for the cancer rates to peak, and why I am urging you to protect yours.

Julius Knapp, from the Federal Communications Commission (FCC), also testified at those Congressional hearings, revealing **"nobody at the agency is competent to evaluate the biology."** The FCC's job is to implement regulations. Although it was invited to testify, the industry's trade group declined, and issued a statement assuring us that there's no scientific basis for any concern about cell phones.

In 2010 Dr. Herberman issued a strong warning:

> There is evidence linking long-term cell phone use to possible adverse health effects including cancer. Although the evidence is still controversial, I am convinced that there are sufficient data to warrant an advisory on cell phone use. A panel of pathologists, oncologists and public health specialists declared that cell phone radiation should be considered a potential human health risk.

A year later, in 2011, Dr. Herberman reported an alarming rise of brain cancer in Scandinavian countries with longer cell phone use:

> Based on the laboratory and epidemiological evidence to date, the grounds for taking precautionary actions to reduce direct exposure to the brain and body from cell phone radiation are stronger than ever.

Yet, there are still health officials, and regulatory agencies, who insist there's no clear evidence of biological effects that could lead to illness or disease. Not so, according to Dr. Magda Havas, who says there are "literally thousands of studies showing serious adverse health effects."

As you may know, studies reporting a range of symptoms and illness from RF exposure go back a long way, and adverse effects occur at a fraction of government standards. *(See page 61.)* In the US and Canada those allowable levels are a whopping 2 to 10 million (microwatts per meter squared). Yes, that is millions, while sleep can be disrupted at .002.

Are your symptoms EMR related? The 4-day Radiation

Not sleeping well, feeling dizzy or having other syı
Wired and wireless radiation exposure could be one reason.
Electro-pollution can make a healthy person feel unwell, and
worsen symptoms in someone with compromised health.
Here's how to try our test.

- Unplug all 2.4, 5.8, or 6.0 GHz cordless phones. Replace them with
  older 900 MHz cordless phones, or even better switch to landlines –
  phones with a corded handset. If you have done away with landline
  service and use mobile phones, you may really benefit from this test,
  and will need to power them off, especially at night.

- To maintain Internet access: a wired router and Ethernet cable, or
  power off your wireless router when not in use, and at night. Disable
  your computers' sending and receiving functions – Airport (MAC)
  – and use airplane mode on all hand-held devices, including iPads.

- Avoid or limit use of all mobile communication devices, talking and
  texting. See our safer use guidelines.

- Unplug wired devices: heating pads, also electric heaters, charging
  stations etc. if they are close to where you sit or sleep.

- An RF meter will test the wireless radiation levels. Test the electrical,
  wired devices with a Gauss meter. You need the correct meter
  (available at www.safelivingtechnologies.ca). Test the levels, reduce
  the exposures – unplugging devices and or replacing them as
  suggested above – then retest.

- Other home sources to disable/unplug: baby monitors, wireless
  security systems, wireless speaker systems, Bluetooth devices,
  microwave ovens.

- At night you can turn off the non-essential circuits in the fuse box

External sources such as your neighbor's Wi-Fi and cordless phones,
cell tower antennas and power lines are not as easy to control. After
4 days, how are you feeling? Tell us at www.radiationrescue.org.

The jury is still out? Or not?

Many experts urge caution, while others, including an industry spokesperson, assure us that there is "no problem as standards have been set with large safety margins". Skeptical?

CNN's Larry King was one of the first high-profile media interviewers to take this issue seriously. He asked the prominent neurosurgeon, Vini Khurana, MD to back up his contention that the danger of cell phones could have far broader health ramifications than asbestos and smoking.

Dr. Khurana's reply:

> I base my statement on the fact, Larry, that at this point in time, there's just over three billion users of cell phones worldwide – half of our world population. And the concern is not just brain tumors, but other health effects including behavioral disturbances, salivary gland tumors, male infertility and microwave sickness syndrome.

Flash forward to Larry King's program when the Interphone study was big news, in 2010. One of his guests, Ellie Marks, became a fierce campaigner when her husband Alan was diagnosed with brain cancer.

Alan writes:

> My medical records were sent to doctors and scientists who determined that my brain tumor was directly attributable to my long term use of my cellular phone. I then heard of other brain tumor patients in the same situation; many much younger, and many no longer alive. I am in real estate and used a cell phone for over 20 years for about 10,000 lifetime hours. I always held my phone

to my right ear and the tumor was on the right side of my brain slightly in front of my ear. Ironic that the very thing that was an integral part of my business to enhance my productivity will kill me.

Ellie Marks is now Director of Government & Public Affairs for Environmental Health Trust (founded by Dr. Davis.) They have a new film, Disconnect, that you should see. Mrs. Marks, who also works with brain cancer victims and their families, tells us why her concern is not just about her husband:

> Alan is just the tip of the iceberg of a pandemic of brain tumors as he used one longer than many Americans. These tumors have a lengthy latency period. What has happened to my husband could easily happen to you, your children, or grandchildren.

Larry King said he would continue to take an interest in this issue. And, astute as ever, he asked the panel about possible cardiac effects. He needs to hear about Dr. Sinatra. I sent a copy of this book to King's office.

Is your family at risk?

One of our readers wrote:

> My husband was almost proud of his 'crackberry' habit. He was getting headaches and dizzy spells, and having trouble sleeping. Your plan has been very helpful. His symptoms have improved and all of us are sleeping much better. I tell anyone who'll listen.

Other concerns: cell phones for safety, video games for activity?

Many parents feel safer knowing their children/teens carry cell phones: you know where they are, and in case of an emergency they can call for help. The kids text, surf the Internet, and play an array of video games.

How many minutes, or hours, a day do your children spend gaming? Do you know?

The games that get them up off the couch and firing away at the screen are great exercise, some believe.

Parents may rationalise it's a real workout and keeps them off the streets. Unbeknownst to most parents, the kids are getting a lot more from this rapid-fire obsession, and many are becoming addicted.

Young people often sleep with cell phones under the pillow to catch that secret call, or text message. Maybe this is why many have trouble getting to sleep and getting up for school? Who wants to sleep when you can twitter?

Dr. Hans Scheiner, a physician with a complementary medicine clinic in Germany told me:

> Children and young people can become physiologically addicted to EMR. So excessive cell phone use and wireless computer games are not just an addictive habit, or a behavioral issue. **EMR opens the blood-brain barrier in the same way as alcohol and drugs.** This can give a feeling of euphoria, and when you try to get them away from the game they'll experience withdrawal symptoms, as you may know if you've tried to reduce your child's computer/gaming time and cell phone use.

Dr. Olle Johansson offers us this concise summary of concern:

> The radiation emitted by mobile phones, and other wireless communication devices, has been shown to damage DNA – leading to possible mutations and cancer development, and is linked to impairments to immune function and neurological diseases and functions – including cognition and behaviour, as well as affecting fertility and reproduction.

This is why I urge you to keep reading through the next section focusing on our children and teens and the health risks facing their wireless generation.

Please remember the plan detailed in this book shows you how to take effective steps to reduce those risks.

Children and Teens on Cell Phones and Cordless Phones

Consider this 2008 study by the Swedish oncologist, Lennart Hardell. Professor Hardell presented new evidence – an analysis of data from one of the biggest cancer risk studies – which shows that:

> children and teenagers are five times more likely to get a certain kind of brain cancer – glioma –

if they begin using cell phones before the age of 20. The extra risk from using cordless phones was found to be almost as high.

When this story was published in the Canadian press, a spokesman for the Canadian Wireless Telecommunications Association told the public:

> Government agencies responsible for compiling and analyzing research – including Health Canada and the World Health Organization – continue to say that the evidence that is out there, that has been reviewed for years and years and years, says there is no demonstrated risk for human health.

Health Canada's response was: "currently we see no scientific reason to consider the use of cell phones as unsafe. There is no convincing evidence of increased risk of disease." (Excerpted from an article by Sarah Schmidt, CanWest News Service)

After the WHO reversed its position on cell phones and related radiation, in 2011, Health Canada issued a cautionary note about those under 18 using mobile phones. Yet few people are making the crucial connection with Wi-Fi, and other wireless devices like iPads.

Hardell's research shows risks also increased with the number of hours of use, the intensity of the phone's power, and the younger the child was when starting to use cell phones. As you know, the children of today will be exposed for decades longer than those of us who got our first mobile in our thirties or forties.

Studies from two other European labs, published in *Physics in Medicine and Biology* (June 7, 2008) show that young children's brains absorb twice as much radiation from a cell phone as the brains of adults.

Children also have thinner skulls and smaller heads than adults, so radiation can penetrate more deeply into the brain – as you see on the book cover that shows an estimation of the absorption of electro-magnetic radiation from a cell phone based on age.

Dr. Davis explains:

> Few parents know that radio-frequency signals reach much more deeply into children's thinner and smaller brains than ours – a fact established through the pioneering work of Professor Om P. Gandhi, the leader of the University of Utah's electrical engineering department.

In 2004, standards became looser, because industry modelers decided to use a new approach – basically doubling the amount of radio-frequency that could reach the brain of an adult and quadrupling that reaching a child's.

The brain of a child doubles in the first two years of life and keeps on developing until their early 20s.

Professor Gandhi no longer works with the cell-phone industry and none of his grandchildren uses a cell phone.

The researcher Dr. George Carlo also pointed out:

From a physiological point of view, children are more susceptible to damage because their cells are differentiating more. The consequences of disrupting cell differentiation are potentially devastating, making it a medical necessity to examine wireless networks in hospitals schools, homes, apartments, and communities.

In 2009, scientists in Europe and the USA were endorsing the BioInitiative Report and calling for world-wide health protection agencies and governments to urgently comply.

The following precautionary actions were proposed:

- **children under 16 should only use cordless and mobile phones in emergencies;**

- **no Wi-Fi, Wi-MAX, or other wireless networking, be placed in homes, schools, or public areas; and**

- conduct independent, widely publicized, frequent audits to ensure base stations do not exceed newly warranted, biologically based standards.

(Professor Johansson. The London Resolution. *Pathophysiology*.)

How can we limit our teens' risky behaviors?

This generation is hard-wired to wireless gadgets. And most of their age group has never been prone to accepting adult advice.

When I was buying a pair of shoes the other day, the young sales person was working his cell phone every few minutes. I felt compelled to ask him if he had heard about health hazards.

The look he gave me wasn't quite the adolescent eye-roll I get from my own children, but it was certainly an expression of disbelief. "Not really interested", he shrugged, "I use this cell phone for everything."

I consulted with Dr. Allison Rees, an expert in parent-teen communication for her advice on how we can approach this challenge; this is coming up with our Action Plan in Strategy 4.

Professor Olle Johansson offers some sobering thoughts:

> Children/teens may be more vulnerable due to the permeability of the skull, and maybe the risk will turn out to be equally large for all ages. But, much more importantly, the effect on children is much more serious for mankind since it hits us at our 'roots' rather than at the 'end-branches', the elderly. As our knowledge stands right now, interaction with fertility, the immune system capacity, shattering of the DNA, or impaired learning and intelligence, will be much more dangerous than the extra cases of cancer.

> Of course, for anyone getting cancer, or being a relative to a cancer victim, they will suffer tremendously, no doubt about that. But, just considering mankind, as a species, we can lose a few, but not everyone.

In 2010 Professor Joel Moskowitz of University of California Berkeley combined information from ALL studies ever done on brain tumors and cell phones and found "consistent evidence that heavy cell phone use (could be as little as 30 minutes daily) for a decade or longer increases brain tumor risk at least 30%."

As you can see, researchers are telling us that with ten years of cell phone use the risk increases anywhere from 30 - 140%. If you also have a mobile device powered on while sleeping, or a cordless phone nearby, the elevated risk may be alarming. How about a bedside Wi-Fi multi-function router/alarm clock/cell phone recharging station?

As concerned as we are about their generation, we must also remember the tragedy of adult brain cancers, as Ellie Marks warns us.

As with most of life's calamities, we assure ourselves, "Not my family."

I have just returned from the standing-room only 'Celebration of Life' of a truly marvelous man and witnessed the tragedy that can strike a man and his young family.

Michael inspired everyone who met him with his humour, modesty and grace – before and after his diagnosis. Even with a scar on the side of his bald head; even when he could no longer walk, he greeted each person, and each situation, with an ear-to-ear smile, radiating kindness. He accepted each day with joyful zest, and always put others first, even toward the end of his journey when he was utterly dependent on them. His wife with such courage, and his two young children with such promise, brought tears to our eyes and somehow hope to our hearts, as they remembered the love and laughter that he brought to them. Michael was 42.

I am sure he and his wife never thought this could happen to their family. We seldom do. And this is what keeps us from taking the proactive steps that could protect us. People often tell me, "Yes, but, my son (husband, daughter) would never give up the cell phone .. on it all the time.. has to have it for work."

There is, however, something suddenly compelling about a positive biopsy. I know from working with cardiac patients how motivating 'a bolt from the blue' like a heart attack can be – at least for the ones who survived. I have talked personally with most of these experts, made a lot of changes in my life, and experienced a lot of benefits. And I have had time to try and come to terms with this, and still find it hard to swallow and digest, so I empathize if you are choking on it.

Why is this chart relevant? To see the massive disparity between the levels considered biologically safe, and the government safety standards that govern the marketplace: A. electrical and B. wireless.

A. ELECTRICAL SOURCES

AC MAGNETIC FIELDS from plugged in devices, household appliances, power lines, ground current issues. Test with a Gauss meter (mG = milligauss).

Building Biology Guidelines (SBM 2008)

1. Sleeping areas

all measures on this page are in milligauss mG	No concern	Slight concern	Severe concern	Extreme concern
	0.2	**0.2-1**	**1 - 5**	**5**

2. Daytime measures (taking into consideration the duration, proximity) should be below **1**

Dr. Martin Blank: biological effects **2 - 5,**

so recommend less than that.

Levels allowed in North America:

833 for the general public,

4,166 for occupational exposure.

Europe: **1,000** for the general public

5,000 for occupational exposure: Source: ICNIRP, 1998.

B. RADIO-FREQUENCY (Wireless) RADIATION SOURCES

Cell tower antennas (masts), Wi-MAX, wireless networks, cell and cordless phones, PDAs, wireless laptops, and other wireless devices.

Test with an RF meter. Make sure your meter's frequency range is high enough. Many meters don't have a high enough range to test newer cordless phones, for example, so you may get a false low reading.

Building Biology Guidelines (SBM 2008)

1. Sleeping areas

measures in microwatts per square meter	No concern	Slight concern	Severe concern	Extreme concern
	< 0.1	**0.1-10**	**10-1000**	**> 1000**

2. Daytime measures should be: **below 10**

Dr. Martin Blank: biological effects occur at: **0.1**

What levels are allowed? 2 - 10 million   Source: ICNIRP, 1998.

Yes, the government standards that regulate radiation emitted from the cell phone held against your head, and the cell tower antenna beside your child's school, are MILLIONS of times away from what is considered biologically safe. This is why assurances such as, "These radiation levels fall within government safety standards," should be questioned, and standards re-evaluated.

In a few pages you will see the RF Guidelines table that shows international levels of this radio-frequency radiation (also known as microwave radiation) from broadcast antennas, cell towers (masts), radar, satellites – wireless communications that now encircle all parts of our planet.

Remember what you just learned about thermal and non-thermal? Some of these international standards are based on the view that as long as the radiation is not powerful enough to cook tissue, then we're just fine. (Or, so their thinking goes.)

I asked the Building Biology environmental consultant, Katharina Gustavs, "just how high are those so-called 'safe' thermal levels?"

Ready for an astronomical number to stretch your comprehension? She answered, "At exposure levels of around 1,000,000,000 (microwatts per sq. meter in the frequency range of 400 MHz to 3 GHz), the eye lens starts to turn opaque; this is referred to as the thermal level."

Yes, that is one billion! So you see why some occupational exposures, including the military in many countries, allow 100,000,000 – why, it's only 1/10th of the allowable thermal level.

If you don't recognize the evidence of biological effects that have been shown to occur at a minuscule 0.1, it can seem that there's 'no problem'. This is the core of the issue, as I see it.

To put this into perspective, I also asked Peter Schlegel, a Swiss civil engineer, "What was the natural background of RF radiation for our ancestors?" I had to pause and count the zeros when he replied, "0.000001 is the estimate."

How's that for an indication of how far we've come in a century of technological development? Schlegel goes on to explain, "this is the cosmic background radiation arriving on earth (source H.-P. Neitzke, ECOLOG Institute, Germany) and it is also a level that living cells respond to."

Knowing this is useful, he tells us, for raising the awareness of the harm we have caused to our environment. However, this low natural level does not exist anymore because it is overpowered by the emissions of our human-made technology.

From 0.000001 to 100,000,000 – anyone have a calculator? One presumes the various species living on this planet had millions of years with the natural background. You can see why so many experts are alarmed at the dramatically increased levels of radiation exposure we're forced to endure now.

I find the recommendation of maximum levels of exposure below 10 for daytime, and below 5 for sleeping, to be very helpful. You need a reliable RF meter to determine these levels – see our Resources section.

The gap between what many scientists consider safe (0.1) and what some organizations/regulations allow (100,000,000) is the same difference in magnitude between the length of a few football fields and the distance from the earth to the sun. Isn't that unbelievable? (See the next page.)

RF Exposure from Cell Towers

ırldwide Limits and Standards in µW/m² (microwatt per square meter)

100,000,000	U.S. Standard C95.1-1966. The first standard limiting exposure to microwaves in the Western world.
10,000,000 to 4,000,000	ICNIRP Guidelines (1998) are based on biological effects of short-term, high-level exposures that cause a rise in temperature, also referred to as thermal effects. Germany (1996), USA (1997), Japan (1997), Switzerland (2000), Australia (2002), Finland (2002), Sweden (2002), UK (2004), Austria (2006), Canada (2009) and many others. Exposure limit depends on frequency of carrier wave (800 MHz to 10 GHz).
2,500,000 to 1,000,000	Belgium law (2001). In 2009 a ruling of the constitutional court concluded that the setting of exposure levels for cell towers lies with the regional not the federal government. Exposure limit depends on frequency of carrier wave (800 MHz to 10 GHz).
100,000	Russia law (2003), China law (1987)
100,000	Italy law (2003): attention level not to be exceeded in sensitive areas.
95,500 to 42,500	Switzerland law (2000): precautionary exposure limit for sensitive areas. Based on the carrier wave frequency of the respective antennas (900 MHz, 1800 MHz, or both), the limit applies to a single transmitter site, including all antennas located on the same cell tower or building. If transmitter sites are spaced closely together, the perimeter of each site (ca. 40-100 m) is defined by the cumulative effective radiated power of all antennas at a given site.
24,000	Belgium: regional law in Brussels (2007), Wallonia (2009), Flanders (2010)
1,000	France: 16 cities chosen by Environment Ministry for pilot project (2010)
1,000	BioInitiative Working Group precautionary recommendation for outdoor environment (2007)
1,000	Salzburg Resolution for sum total of GSM (2000)
170	Seletun Consensus Statement – a precautionary recommendation (2010)
100	BioInitiative Working Group precautionary recommendation for indoor environment (2007)
100	BUND (Friends of the Earth Germany) recommendation for hazard protection (2008)
1	BUND (Friends of the Earth Germany) recommendation for precautionary protection (2008)
1	Health Department, Federal State of Salzburg, Austria precautionary recommendation for indoor environment of sum total of GSM (2002)
< 0.1 **No concern**	**Building Biology Evaluation Guidelines** (SBM 2008) specifically designed for sleeping areas and empirically established on the basis of many thousands of individual cases, including EHS sufferers. This precautionary threshold level of 0.1 is generally adopted by all Building Biology environmental consultants who conduct professional RF surveys in homes, at workplaces, for EHS sufferers.

0.000001 Natural background – mostly this low natural level does not exist anymore.

Prepared by Katharina Gustavs, 2012 Printed here with permission.

How is this massive safety margin gap affecting our families? Do we even know? I have a cousin in a navy radar unit; it is chilling to realize the extreme levels he is being exposed to onboard ship. Now that you know about this measurement of RF radiation let's take a look at some of the levels we may be exposed to.

Katharina Gustavs reports on this RF (radio-frequency):

> For the sum total of the background RF radiation level in urban areas, you can find in the literature levels ranging from one hundred (microwatts per sq. meter) all the way up to a few thousand, or even into the ten thousands, depending on how close the next base station is located.

Risks from Cell Tower Antennas / Masts In Your Community?

A German study reported that living within 400 meters (1300 ft) of two antennas over 10 years increased rates of cancer three fold. Living closer than that, they warned, the risk could be 100 fold. In Israel, a Tel Aviv University study also showed an increased cancer risk with proximity to antennas. Researchers in Australia, the UK and Italy found significant increase in leukemia. Many advocacy groups are fighting the installations of cell towers/masts in their communities. You can find a group in your area, or start your own. (Check out the Index for our Statement of Accountability – a useful tool in this fight.)

In the US, the proliferation at www.antennasearch.com will alarm you, as will the rate at which transmitters are installed close to your home, child's school or hospital. Why are we allowing these so close? Outdated safety standards. Regulatory inertia. Talk to your school, other parents, and local representatives. At www.electromagnetichealth.org there is an important report "The BRAG™ Antenna Ranking of Schools" by Dr. Magda Havas who is working tirelessly, and effectively, for us all.

Proximity to cell tower antennas/masts/base stations

Many experts report that harmful biological effects occur at so called "safe" levels. The neuroscientist Dr Sarah Starkey sent us this update:

> In 2010 Dr Khurana reported in the *International Journal of Occupational and Environmental Health* that 8 out of 10 published epidemiological studies reported increased adverse neurobehavioral symptoms or cancer in populations living **within 500 meters (1640 feet)** of cell tower antennas (mobile phone base stations). Also in 2010, Balmori found developmental abnormalities and 90% mortality of tadpoles (compared to 4.2% mortality for those screened from the radiation) after two months of living near a cell tower antenna. In the journal *Pathophysiology* (2009), Otitoloju reported developmental sperm abnormalities from mice living near an antenna for six months and many associations between this proximity and damage to wildlife. The Stewart Report, commissioned by the UK Government in 2000, recommended that the beam of greatest intensity of this radiation should not fall on a school's grounds or buildings.

In 2011 a Brazilian study led by engineer Adilza Dode, PhD also linked cell tower radiation with cancer deaths among people living within the same distance – 500 meters (1640 feet). Dr. Dode warns that emission limits are not based on health criteria, but upon industrial, economic and technological criteria. A study by Dr. Henry Lai and Blake Levitt, published by the National Research Council Press, recommended **"keep cell towers far from people"** and cautioned that proximity to Wi-Fi, Wi-MAX, and SmartGrids also increases people's cancer risks.

It's not just cancer; a long-term study from Rimbach Germany, published in 2011, showed harmful effects on neurotransmitters – electric impulses in our brain. This is a concern for us, at every age!

Strategy I. Know the Evidence

Risks at your school?

OMG page! (handwritten)

A mom wrote that her school principal reassured her that, "Th[ ] in the school were well within the government safety standards." I told her about the research and suggested she show it to the school, and other parents. Who better to fight for our children than us, the parents?

Some RF risks in your own home?

While it is essential that we have some comprehension of the exposures in our external environment, and that we make our voices heard, we should also be mindful of our exposures inside. Building Biology consultant, Peter Sierck, comments:

> We see many people fighting the installation of cell towers (masts) and going home where they have wireless routers and cordless phones which constantly radiate without being in use, microwave ovens, and often mobile phones.

OMG (handwritten)

Common Exposure Levels (all in microwatts per sq. meter)

Let's take a look at some measures taken by Gustavs and others.

Wireless Internet access An average-powered home wireless router within one foot (30 cm) – 30,000, within 10 ft (3 meters) – 3,000

A cordless phone (5.8 or DECT 6.0) within one foot (30 cm) – 200,000, within 10 ft (3 meters) – 2,000

A microwave oven in use (new, not defective) within one foot (30 cm) – 10,000-1,000,000, within 10 ft (3 meters) – 1,500

In an average 2-3 bedroom home that has a wireless router and at least one cordless phone: (KG) "If the cordless phone is in the bedroom, the person in bed may be exposed to 20,000 all night long, and in the kitchen maybe only 200. Again, the router at the desk may expose the computer user to 20,000, while in the living room next door you may have 1,000 and in the bedroom further away – 100."

Cognitive Impairment, Cardiac Effects and Cancer Risks?

After the memorial service for her husband – her high school sweetheart – who died of a brain tumor, the widow was consumed with grief. Now she is getting angry. He was a commercial pilot who used a cell phone for many years. One year she gave him one of those in-the-ear wireless bluetooth headsets, hoping it would help. She discovers that air crews' EMR exposure, including cosmic radiation, has caused cancer concerns for many years; and that now there is more exposure in the skies. She reads that a group of European physicians have issued an urgent medical alert about cell phones and wireless Internet onboard. Evidently, it was ignored.

The physicians had warned that this radiation can affect cognitive function and reduce reaction time – crucial factors in aviation – and put the crew at greater cancer risk. She used to assume that the strictly controlled aviation industry, and other regulatory agencies, were being vigilant about the health and safety of the flight crews and passengers. Now she is not so sure.

Smart Meters, Smart Grids and Smart Appliances

Are you suspicious yet of technologies labelled "smart"? The health concerns are *not* just about one Smart Meter, but hubs of them in high-density dwellings, the prospect of billions of them around the world, and their powerful wireless Smart Grid/Wi-MAX networks. Smart Meters send out frequent bursts of data (energy consumption readings) from your house to your neighbor's, then to the power company. Electro-sensitive people, and others, could suffer from this involuntary exposure. The emission levels "meet government standards and are too low to cause harm," officials declare. Let's ask some hard questions: Where is the evidence that this radiation, re-classified in 2011 by the WHO as "possibly carcinogenic", will not be harmful? What agency is monitoring our accumulated dose of exposure? Why are you forging ahead, when some utilities are removing Smart Meters? (Due to health concerns, in the fall of 2011, California's PG&E was 'quietly' replacing wireless Smart Meters with analog/wired ones – the safe option.) And is your agency/company insured for health claims?

Fiber optics is the best choice for data communication, according to many technical and health experts. This system has many benefits. The data are sent along fiber optic cables, using pulses of light – safe – and also secure as this is a closed system. There are no radiation emissions blasting through space and all living creatures. Fiber optics can deliver Internet access and other communication data. Initially, this may be more expensive, but consider the health savings – see page 333.

Natural World at Risk

As we mentioned earlier, electro-pollution affects all life forms, not just us humans.

Where have all the bees gone?

With disbelief and mounting concern, the old beekeeper notices the bees have disappeared again.

As he stands in his field inspecting the empty hives, he looks up and sees the cell tower antennas glaring down at him from the peak of the hill nearby. "Such unsightly things", he grumbles.

Half a world away, in an English village, an elderly church custodian is blissfully unaware of the cell antenna in his neighborhood; it is embedded in the shiny new metal cross, high upon the church tower.

He has been watching for the return of the barn swallows, as he has done for years. Where are the birds, he wonders?

Why are they not making it back here?

Evidently, the adverse effects of disrupting the intra-cellular whispering that Dr. Adey described are not limited to the human species. Some researchers say EMR is also disrupting the natural navigation abilities of whales, birds and bees.

Strategy 1. Know the Evidence

Dr. Carlo offered this explanation:

BEES

> The disappearance of bees – Colony Collapse Disorder – has occurred concurrently on four continents within a very short time frame. This hardly ever happened before and its implications are dire: how will our crops become pollinated? What will become of our food supply?
>
> If the reason was biological or chemical, as some say, there would be a pattern of epidemic spread – we would be able to trace the source, similar to the spread of SARS a few years ago. That is not the case.
>
> The colony collapse has hit each continent at roughly the same time. That would mean the cause hit the continents at the same time, as well. Mobile phones meet that criterion.
>
> The information-carrying radio waves from these, and other, wireless devices, disrupt inter- and intra-cellular communication in most species.
>
> Therefore, it is biologically plausible that the bees, exposed to this radiation, cannot find their way back to the hive, and starve.

Agriculture at Risk

Perhaps, we should consider this quote from Albert Einstein, "No more bees, no more pollination ... no more humans!"

It's Not Just the Bees

In 1971 William Kenton of Cornell University studied the effect of electro-magnetic fields on birds' ability to migrate:

> ...with 1-gauss (electrically-charged) magnets attached to their heads the birds couldn't find their way home. Each bird without magnets faultlessly navigated the 150 miles ...and fluttered in like a helicopter to a perfect landing.

Arthur Firstenberg wrote in *The Ecologist* in June 2004:

> Canadian researchers working with parakeets, chickens, pigeons and seagulls reported that these birds avoided microwave fields (EMR) if they could, and collapsed within seconds if they couldn't. Many years later, Alfonso Martínez carefully documented the decline and disappearance of white storks, house sparrows, and free-tailed bats from the vicinity of cellular phone base stations.

More than forty-five years ago, Rachel Carson wrote:

> Over increasingly large areas of the US, spring now comes unheralded by the return of the birds, and the early mornings are strangely silent where they were once filled with the beauty of bird song.

More than 100 years ago, Anton Chekhov warned:

> Human beings have been endowed with reason and creative power. But they have been more destructive than creative. Forests are disappearing, rivers are drying up, and wildlife is becoming extinct.

Before a radar station in Latvia was shut down at the end of the Cold War, a co-ordinated effort was made to determine whether the station had any environmental impact.

Even at extremely low levels of exposure, researchers found these effects: smaller growth rings in trees, premature ageing in pine needles, (a factor in raging wildfires in heavily populated, high-EMR areas?) and they found chromosome damage in cows.

And Wolfgang Volkrodt linked forest die-back to microwave radiation rather than acid rain.

Also in Germany, Löscher and Käs documented illness in dairy cows caused by cell towers. You don't have to be a dairy farmer to realize the serious implications of this.

Wildlife and Domestic Animals at Risk

Wildlife biologist Alfonso Balmori, PhD of Valladolid, Spain reported that:

> **Electromagnetic radiation is a form of environmental pollution which may hurt wildlife.** Phone masts (cell towers) located in their living areas are irradiating continuously some species that could suffer long-term effects, like reduction of their natural defenses, deterioration of their health, problems in reproduction and reduction of their useful territory through habitat deterioration.
>
> Therefore microwave and radio-frequency pollution constitutes a potential cause for the decline of animal populations and deterioration of health of plants living near phone masts.

Nature at Risk

Dr. Ulrich Warnke of the University of Saarland, in Germany cautioned a recent conference organized by Radiation Research in the UK that electro-smog was "disrupting nature on a massive scale".

Dr. Warnke went on to say:

> Today, unprecedented exposure levels from numerous wireless technologies interfere with the natural information system and functioning of humans, animals, and plants. The consequences of this development, which have already been predicted by critics for many decades, cannot be ignored anymore. Bees and other insects vanish; birds avoid certain places, and become disorientated at others.
>
> Humans suffer from functional impairments and diseases. And insofar as the latter are hereditary, they will be passed on to next generations as pre-existing defects.

> Now that we have investigated some of the evidence of harm from the electro-pollution which surrounds us, I must pose these questions: How much more evidence do we need before taking a course of action? And where are those who are charged with public health safety?

Agencies Passing the Buck?

Alasdair Philips, the Director of Powerwatch, is realistic:

> I am a practising engineer and scientist who did amateur radio transmitter work. I thought wireless was brilliant. I now believe that the mistake we are making will have much more serious long-term effects than either smoking tobacco, or asbestos. Wireless is one of the few boom industries today, and one that brings governments massive tax revenues. So neither governments, nor the wireless industries, want any official word of precaution to be issued – however gently it is worded.

> There is good evidence of some harm (at least) and we should be warning people not to use such technologies when other, less invasive, ones are available that often (like Ethernet wired networks v.s. wLAN/Wi-Fi) actually perform better, and do not expose people to radio-frequency radiation. Why can't we warn people about the dangers of excessive exposures to relatively low levels of radio-frequency radiation. To use caution.

Economics Over Public Health?

Relying on government and public health officials to safeguard our wellbeing has seldom been prudent. Whenever I hear an official proclaim, "there is no conclusive evidence", I vow to find more brave souls like the feisty Canadian physician Dr. Francis Kelsey. She was working in the US and prevented the use of thalidomide by pregnant women. Canada and many other countries didn't heed her wise use of the precautionary principle. We know the tragic cost of their negligence: thousands of babies born with birth defects.

Unfortunately, the dispute about the regulations controlled by ICNIRP, the World Health Organization, and various federal government agencies, continues. This controversy is not very helpful when you're wondering about that powerful multi-purpose PDA.

I heard one expert warn that these powerful new multi-task phones are getting close to thermal levels. Is some government agency monitoring this? Or monitoring the people getting sick, or those who are dying? I discovered that the European Union's main environmental watchdog, the EEA, and the BioInitiative Working Group – an international team of scientists, researchers and public health policy professionals – were both warning that government standards are woefully inadequate. Truth is, they're irrelevant, according to the BioInitiative Report.

(Check out www.healthandenvironment.org for information, and for the BioInitiative Report go to www.bioinitiative.org.)

In 2010, Dr. Louis Slesin commented on these regulations:

> The Finnish Radiation and Nuclear Safety Authority recommended that parents limit children's use of mobile phones and, on the same day, the French government announced a series of environmental health proposals, which include a ban on advertising that promotes the use of cell phones among those under 12. In contrast to all this activity, the lackadaisical approach of the International Commission on Non-Ionizing Radiation Protection (ICNIRP) is striking. Some 40 countries, many of which have only limited expertise in RF radiation health effects, look to the Commission for advice. **Yet, ICNIRP has been silent for ten long years. Their last standards on RF exposures were published in 1998.** How long could it take to write a simple statement urging caution?

Dr. Slesin gave us an update for this 2012 edition:

> It's not easy to reach unanimous agreement on anything to do with cell phone radiation. But IARC (the International Agency for Research on Cancer– part of the World Health Organization) nearly pulled it off. In May, more than two dozen scientists and doctors from 14 countries – a group IARC Director Christopher Wild called 'the world's leading experts' – issued a joint statement that cell phone and other types of radiofrequency (RF) and microwave radiation might cause cancer.
>
> A month later the international regulator – ICNIRP – announced that its epidemiologists believe that cell phones are safe. They conceded that they couldn't be certain, though they sounded as if they were nearly there.

A European gathering was held in Brussels in 2009. The Mobile Manufacturers Forum (a lobby organization) presented reasons why it believes its members are sufficiently protected from criticism and potential litigation – because products (i.e. mobile phones) comply for the most part with ICNIRP safety limits.

David Gee, one of the authors of the BioInitiative Report, warned:

> Mobile phone manufacturers will not be able to claim immunity if, in ten years or so, it is determined that use of mobile phones causes brain cancer or other illness. The mobile phone manufacturers are forewarned now, and simply saying 'but we were in compliance with ICNIRP safety limits' will not be sufficient reason for ignoring the growing evidence.

US Federal Regulations – Protecting Americans?

Professor Devra Davis, the noted epidemiologist comments:

> The agency that offers recommendations on cell-phone emissions in the U.S. – the Federal Communications Commission – doesn't employ a single health expert. The standards the FCC adopts are based on advice given by outside experts, many of whom work directly for the cell-phone industry.
>
> The Food and Drug Administration lacks the authority to set standards for cell phones and can only act if a phone is shown to release hazardous signals.

Yes, this is a lot of information to absorb. By the way, I hope you are not reading this on your wirelessly-connected mobile.

We've seen how the regulations are not protecting us. As you read through this, please remember that help is on the way.

Scientists including Dr. Davis and Dr. Blank, and dedicated advocates including the publisher Dr. Louis Slesin, are highly effective in educating people about this issue, and media coverage is increasing. As people wake up, legislators in the US, and other countries, will be forced to take action.

Your Assessment So Far?

How are you doing in your assessment of this issue? As you can see, I have formed mine and sincerely believe that we are putting ourselves and our loved ones at risk, and I have taken steps to protect my family. But it is *your* view that is most relevant here. I hope this book is helpful.

Are the wireless or insurance industries alerting customers?

Do you read the fine print on your cell phone contract?

Who does? But you might check to see if you are agreeing not to participate in any class action lawsuits, or have missed safety precautions.

I heard that after 2002 the insurance industry began excluding health risk claims from the product liability policies that they were selling to the mobile phone industry. Is this true?

In other words, it appears that insurance underwriters such as Lloyds of London may have refused to insure cell phone manufacturers against health-related claims. Remember how few class action suits it took to seriously damage the asbestos and the breast implant industries?

We are told that since as much as 30% of retirement fund shares are invested in the telecommunications industry, a series of class action suits could be disastrous to retirees, and to the already bruised western economies. And, of course, to the telecom industry.

You might also carefully read the information that came with your cell phone or PDA to see how far away from your head they recommend you hold this device. If held against the head, many exceed government standards. Warning: It is in tiny print. We've been fairly warned. Or have we?

So Who is Taking Action?

As you know, Europe and the UK are more densely populated than most of North America, and with that comes a correspondingly thick cloud of electro-smog. In some cities the ambient levels of radiation are so high that virtually everyone is being exposed, even those choosing not to use cell phones. There are reports that in many countries upwards of 5 – 10% of the population is already experiencing related symptoms, so that may be why the wireless safety issue is getting more attention from legislators. The public's mobile phone fixation does not appear to have been quelled, however. Just stroll the streets of any city.

There are more encouraging signs that the tide is turning: some agencies are listening to the independent scientists urging them to bring the safety regulations in line with the science.

Many parent and consumer groups are demanding product safety and accountability – the wellbeing of people over profit. Proactive people all over the world are deciding *not* to wait for the indisputable smoking gun before taking precautions, especially with young, developing brains. And while most governments are lagging behind, others are opting for the precautionary principle. What are you choosing for your family?

In the US

In September 2009 I attended an international conference on cell phones and health, organized by Dr. Devra Davis in Washington, DC. One afternoon, we attended a US Senate Hearing on this subject, requested by Senator Arlen Specter of Pennsylvania and chaired by Sen. Tom Harkin of Iowa. Sen. Mark Prior of Arkansas also attended.

A scientist (speaking for the wireless industry?) caused a stir in the gallery with the claim, "The current scientific evidence does not demonstrate that wireless causes cancer, or other adverse health effects."

(Flashback: one after the other, a line up of Big Tobacco executives assures a Senate hearing, "Senator, nicotine is *not* addictive.")

It was captivating to witness the eminent scientists Drs. Henry Lai, Om Gandhi, Martin Blank and Leif Salford in attendance. During a discussion between the panel of presenters and the senators about Dr. Lai's seminal work on DNA damage, I wanted to leap up and shout, "Dr. Lai is here. Let's ask him about the evidence."

At the closing, Senator Harkin commented, "I found this really very interesting and very challenging, and I can assure you we are going to do some follow-up on this."

I am grateful to Dr. Davis for her clear and compelling testimony at this Senate hearing, and for her book, *Disconnect – The Truth About Cell Phone Radiation* (Plume, 2011).

Other US legislators are responding. Christiane Tourtet, BA, Founder of International MCS/EMS Awareness, brought this issue to Connecticut Governor M. Jodi Rell and Colorado Governor Bill Ritter, Jr.

In 2010, Maine Rep. Andrea Boland presented a bill that would have required cell phones to carry warning labels, like tobacco. It was voted down. San Francisco Mayor Gavin Newsom, undaunted by industry pressure, passed a bill which requires retailers to post cell phone radiation levels. (See page 140 about this specific absorption rate, SAR.) "This will protect the consumers' right to know," said Mayor Newsom, "and encourage the redesign of devices to function at lower radiation levels." California Senator Mark Leno introduced a similar state bill.

And Congressman Dennis Kucinich (D-OH), who has met with Ellie Marks, introduced a bill to create a new national research program to study cell phone risks, to require an update of the SAR, and to grant a consumer's right to know by providing warning labels. He declared,

"We need a first-class research program to give us answers. Obviously, cell phone companies should not be the ones making decisions for us."

We owe a debt of gratitude to legislators who show political bravery. Please contact your representatives and ask what they know about this issue. Without overwhelming them, offer the evidence about wireless radiation and human health, with references, and ask for a response. Best to avoid an angry, alarmist tone, even if you are feeling that way.

Also in 2010, the President's Cancer Panel, which had received extensive information from Eileen O'Connor of EM Radiation Research Trust, issued its report, "Reducing Environmental Cancer Risk."

In Microwave News, Dr. Slesin summarizes that report:

> The Panel's #1 recommendation is: 'A precautionary, prevention-oriented approach should replace current reactionary approaches to environmental contaminants in which human harm must be proven before action is taken to reduce or eliminate exposure.
>
> It is vitally important to recognize that children are far more susceptible to damage from environmental carcinogens.'
>
> Martha Linet, the head of the Radiation Epidemiology Branch at the National Cancer Institute says: 'The most urgent issue that we need to address is whether children or adolescents using cell phones are at increased risk.'

In Canada

Dr. Keith Martin, MP, MD – a physician and Member of Parliament – (now retired) called for government action, "Canada needs to engage in an independent assessment of the effects of electro-magnetic radiation on human health. Recent research has created significant concerns."

Carol Hughes, MP, was involved with the federal Health Committee hearings held in 2010, and has spoken out strongly, "Health Canada must tell Canadians the full story when it comes to microwave irradiation of children. What we're doing by exposing them to all day Wi-Fi in school is really a big experiment, with unknowing volunteers."

And in 2009, Mayor David Saunders of Colwood, British Columbia, signed the Porto Alegre Resolution, becoming the first city in North America to support this call for the precautionary principle.

In the UK

The Leader of the UK Green Party, Caroline Lucas, MEP, said:

> We need a moratorium on mast installations (cell towers) until there is sufficient independent evidence to guarantee their safety. This approach, in keeping with the precautionary principle, is in marked contrast to the position adopted by industry and government which assumes they are safe until proven otherwise.

Another member of parliament in the UK, Dr. Ian Gibson, MP, is supportive. Dr. Gibson's academic training in biology and genetics gives him a special understanding. And some school officials are taking action and have independently decided to remove wireless radiation.

In Europe

In 2007, after an extensive study, the EEA – Europe's top environmental agency – called for immediate steps to reduce exposure from cell towers and other wireless radiation, warning that delay may result in a health crisis more serious than AIDS, and those caused by smoking, pesticides, asbestos and leaded gasoline.

In its report this agency advises us about standards around the world:

> Safety limits set for radiation are thousands of times too lenient, and an official British report concluded that it could not rule out the development of cancers. The EEA's initiative will increase pressure on governments and public health bodies to take precautionary action over the electro-magnetic radiation from rapidly expanding new technologies. The German government is advising its citizens to use wired Internet connections instead of Wi-Fi, and corded landlines instead of mobile phones.

In 2008 the European Parliament voted by 522 to 16 to urge ministers across Europe to bring in stricter limits for exposure to radiation from mobile and cordless phones, wireless Internet and other devices, stating: "The limits on exposure to electro-magnetic fields which have been set for the general public are obsolete."

In 2009 these same European parliamentarians took another step, passing a major resolution that antennas, mobile phone towers and other EMR-emitting devices should be placed a specific distance away from schools, retirement homes and health institutions, and consumers, especially children.

At a 2009 conference held in Brussels, Andrzej Rys, MD, Director of Public Health for the European Commission, spoke of the need for continuing progress on new, biologically-based exposure standards, and implementing precautionary strategies.

In 2011 the Parliamentary Assembly Council of Europe recommended that "for children in general, and particularly in schools and classrooms, preference should be given to wired Internet connections, and the use of mobile phones by schoolchildren on school premises should be strictly regulated." Sound advice. Is it being followed in your school?

Some European member states have taken action. Wireless Internet has already been banned in public schools in Frankfurt, Germany, and Austria's Medical Association is pressing for a similar ban.

Several libraries in Paris have removed their wireless Internet networks due to health concerns. And, in 2009 it was announced that France was prohibiting cell phone use in elementary schools.

Herouville-St.Clair, France is the world's first municipality to remove wireless from schools and public buildings. Citing the precautionary principle, Mayor Rudolphe Thomas declared, "Our job is to protect people's health. And, certainly we are *not* willing to gamble with our children's health." This is a good investment. They are also investing in a Wi-Fi-free fiber optics network – the way of the future!

And the Mayor of the City of Oullins decreed that new mobile phone masts could not be built within 100 meters of schools or day care centers. Also in France, the Senate moved toward banning cell phone use in schools, by children up to about age 14. What's more, the phone companies are required to make sure the electro-magnetic emissions, within this protected zone, do not exceed the low levels recommended in the BioInitiative Report.

A district court also cited the precautionary principle when it issued an injunction stopping a French telecom company from installing cell phone antennas on a hotel, 15 meters from an apartment building in Paris. The plaintiffs argued that the antenna would beam radiation directly into their apartment bedroom. The judgment said, "Even if present scientific knowledge does not enable us to determine precisely the impact of electro-magnetic radiation when it penetrates the communal parts of the building, there exists a risk that cannot be ignored of repercussions on the state of health of the residents who live in it." Health agencies in several nations – Switzerland, Germany, Israel, France, the United Kingdom, and Finland – have issued warnings to limit cell phone use, particularly by children.

It's not all success stories. Industry pressure is strong. In 2000, Salzburg, Austria, with the guidance of renowned physician, Dr. Gerd Oberfeld, had set limits based on biological effects. However, only one of the operators observed the agreement, for a short time, then withdrew.

And the Liechtenstein Parliament had confirmed its intention to restrict exposure from mobile telecom base stations to the BioInitiative Report's recommended levels, by 2013, in sensitive areas such as homes, workplaces, schools, hospitals and public buildings. The wireless companies threatened to pull out, saying the new rules would make it impossible to be financially viable. In a referendum, initiated by industry, the voters rejected the proposed reduction of the safety standard value.

Scientists are Also Taking Action

As you may know, scientists prefer to take an unbiased approach to their research and present their papers within the scientific community. In this case, the recognition that there is growing evidence of harm has brought many of them to speak out publicly.

Elizabeth Kelley, MA directs the International Commission for Electromagnetic Safety (ICEMS), composed of many concerned scientists whose research findings indicate that industry driven exposure standards are not protective and are calling for nations to adopt biologically-based standards.

The International EMF Alliance (IEMFA), a global consortium whose members cover a diversity of medical, scientific and related disciplines, provides health-oriented information and advice.

Citizens are Taking Action

USA

To advance public health policy on this ever-increasing public exposure, The EMR Policy Institute – led by Janet Newton and Diana Warren – focuses its activities on the recommendations to protect human health set forth in the BioInitiative Report.

The Environmental Working Group is a nonprofit organization based in Washington, DC. Their mission includes protecting children, babies, and infants in the womb from health problems attributed to toxic contaminants, including electro-pollution, as well as federal policies.

Center for Safer Wireless is an expanding national non-profit group, founded by health advocate Christine Hoch, to enhance the public's understanding of the safety concerns about wireless products.

Another effective voice is the dedicated Camilla Rees, the founder of ElectromagneticHealth.org and co-author with Dr. Havas of *Public Health SOS: The Shadow Side of the Wireless Revolution*.

Here is an inspiring example of what a grandmother can do: when her grandsons became ill, and EMR exposure was a factor, Joanne Mueller started an organization aptly named, Guinea Pigs "R" Us.

Canada

Martin Weatherall and the Canadian Initiative to Stop Wireless, Electric, and Electromagnetic Pollution (WEEP) educate the public, and provide help for electro-sensitive people.

In British Columbia advocates are making great strides forward: Sharon Noble, founder of CAUSE, was a leading force in getting Colwood to recognize electro-sensitivity and adopt the Porto Alegre Resolution. Una St Clair-Moniz and her group, Citizens for Safe Technology (CST), were also successful in educating local legislators. In October 2010, the Council of White Rock BC voted to request Health Canada to re-evaluate the government's regulations – Safety Code 6.

The UK

Alasdair Philips (Powerwatch), an electrical engineer with extensive knowledge of EMR, is a strong voice for reason and a Contributing Expert for this book. He has advised the British government.

Eileen O'Connor, Director of EM Radiation Research Trust, is a founding Board Member of the EMF Alliance, and an effective voice educating governments and health agencies, including the European Union, British Parliament and WHO.

Sarah Dacre (ES-UK), and others, are educating the public, and providing information and support for those with electro-sensitivity.

WiredChild is a charity run by a concerned parents raising awareness of risks to children from mobile phones and other wireless technology. And Mast Sanity campaigns against the unsafe placement of masts.

Europe

HESE (Human Ecological Social Economical Project) is an international group of researchers and advocates, many with ES/EHS.

France

PRIARTéM (Pour une réglementation des Implantations d'Antennes Relais de Téléphonie Mobile) helps citizens fight for protection of their health. Next-Up is another effective non-governmental group.

Sweden

Sweden has support for people with electro-sensitivity and several of the world's leading researchers are Swedish. In Gothenburg, Anne-Li Karlsson and Jennie Öberg, with others, built a radiation-blocking Faraday cage, in the shape of a house, to show sources of radiation.

Norway

Citizens' Radiation Protection is a group founded by Sissel Halmøy, MS. She is also Founder and Chair of the International EMF Alliance.

Australia

EMFacts Consultancy, founded in 1994 by Don Maisch, PhD, has published a range of reports and papers. And three neurosurgeons, Drs. Vini Khurana, Charles Teo, and Richard Bittar, are speaking out with their concerns about brain tumours and mobile phone use. The Australasian College of Nutritional and Environmental Medicine has published a number of papers. And EMR Australia is a consumer advocacy group alerting people about the growing concerns.

New Zealand

Oururah NZ provides information to people on the adverse health effects of antennas and mobile phones with an extensive website. Another active group in New Zealand is Ban The Tower.

These are just some of the citizens' groups who are taking action. The Resources section has the websites of these groups, and more.

Microwave News has a detailed list of organizations around the globe. Yes, we know we are fighting against the tide (and waves!)

We can turn this around

Never underestimate the impact of a grass-roots groundswell, or the protective dedication of parents and grandparents, when we realize our children are in danger. We are not so blinded by shiny new electronics, convenience or profits. We *will* get regulations based on the biological effects, and be successful in our awareness campaign.

And we will discover more friends of the future. These are rare in the wireless maelstrom, but shining examples of what we can achieve.

Waking Up

If you're still reading along here with me, I imagine you're getting a good sense of the concern. I realize this first section throws a lot at you. Please don't put this book down now! There is also progress in the evidence, and the many things you can do. With any wake-up call, including the morning alarm (not, I hope, from your cell phone), it is tempting to roll over and go back to sleep. Let's keep going for all those we love.

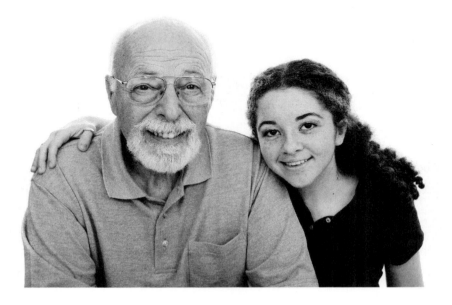

Some days, I wish I could walk away from this. Then I see a child pressing a hot pink cell phone against her head, a baby in the arms of someone on a cordless phone, or a person lying on a heating pad.

As you know, many people will have to mull this over; others act quickly.

A take-action kind of mom I know got the message about wireless networks right away, "That's it, I'm ripping that router out of our house and going back to our Ethernet connection. It worked fine."

I did point out that the risk is not yet a scientific certainty. She shot back, "With my children, I don't wait for that."

A grandmother also woke up on the spot, "My son put this wireless thing in my house so he could get his email in the living room. What about their home and my grandchildren? Their bedrooms are full of electrical things. I'm calling him right now."

Another parent, whose child has autism symptoms, spontaneously hugged me when I told her that many of these children were thriving in a low-EMR environment, and about a new study with promising results, which we will discuss later on.

Let's not fall into the extremes of ignoring this, or becoming anxious. We have a plan that works, and we must not forget that there are many health-enhancing electro-magnetic fields. Some are known as life force, chi – the healing energy in us, and around us. We generate our own bio-electrical field, which is inherently in harmony with the energies that surround us in the natural world. To reconnect with these is another good reason to push back from the computer and step outside.

Acupuncturists, and many other practitioners of energy medicine, work with our inner energetic flow to encourage our innate self-healing mechanisms.

In later strategies, we will look at these natural energies and the healing benefits of these traditions. The key, as in many things, is balance. We can withstand a certain amount of EMR and other toxicity, as long as our innate wellbeing is not overwhelmed. Our basic healthiness and ability to heal are miraculous beyond measure, and can be supported in ways we will discuss. Every contributor to this book is supporting you.

We industrious human beings created this electro-pollution, and we can reverse it. We will meet this Radiation Rescue Challenge™, for all of our children.

In the next section we turn to the crucial strategy of taking stock.

The benefits of this include knowing how much EMR exposure you, and your family, are dealing with on a daily basis; how this may be affecting you, and symptoms and medical conditions. Then we look at safer options for your living, working and travelling environments.

First, I'd like you to read about a teen with electro-sensitivity and understand why we are fighting for him, and for all the others.

Is your child being affected by wireless radiation? A mom's story:

Our 17 year old son was complaining of headaches; an inability to focus; exhaustion even after a long sleep; stomach pains and nausea; clumsiness, and weak legs. Many specialists, from allergists to neurologists, found nothing. Running with his gym class, he'd get sudden pains in his head and nausea – at the same place on the run. (Close to two cell towers, as it turns out.) He always felt really good in remote and unpopulated mountains. No symptoms there.

About a year ago, a building biologist did some testing in our home and suggested he might be electro-sensitive. We had Wi-Fi and cordless 6.0 phones, including one by his bed. His symptoms worsened about a month after we got these 'conveniences'. Was there a connection I wondered?

One evening he was on the computer, near the Wi-Fi router, slouched over his work and struggling with homework. Without his knowing, I unplugged the router. He sat up straight – like a puppet being pulled up on strings. After 15 minutes, secretly, I plugged the router back in. He slumped back down. This was enough proof for me. We removed every radiating device. (Amazingly, my heart palpitations, and my husband's arthritis symptoms, also improved.)At the end of this summer, our son was full of energy. Now he is back at school and has gone from a clear-thinking, sociable, happy teenager into a foggy-brained zombie. He says he feels isolated. There are Wi-Fi routers at his school – for staff use only – one is in his English class. In that class he can only do a few questions in an hour. While at home, he can easily complete 23 questions in half an hour. I have asked the school administration if cabled options could replace the Wi-Fi. They defer to School District policy, which defers to government exposure standards.

Strategy 2 Know Your Risks

THIS SELF-ASSESSMENT QUESTIONNAIRE will help you identify:

- the sources of radiation from wireless and wired devices;

- the symptoms and conditions that may be related.

Remember, just because there are no symptoms it does *not* mean there are no adverse effects.

Do you know where you are on this spectrum, and what to do?

- exposure without symptoms;

- mild to moderate symptoms;

- electro-sensitivity;

- electro-hypersensitivity;

- electro-allergy;

- other serious medical conditions.

And in this step you learn the basics of electro-magnetic radiation – a simple and accurate primer including the difference between wired and wireless radiation. This will help you understand how to take steps that will decrease – not increase – your risk.

See Strategy 2 for more details.

Difficulty sleeping, headaches, increased stress, trouble concentrating, dizziness, impaired immune systems, food allergies and chemical sensitivities can all be connected with EMR exposure. Hans Scheiner, MD

Strategy 2. Know Your Risks

- throughout each day, we are exposed to artificial EMR;

- these levels have been shown to have adverse biological effects;

- this exposure now begins in utero;

- there is a range of related symptoms and health conditions;

- many medical tests and treatments expose us to EMR;

- millions of people around the world are affected by new conditions: electro-sensitivity or electro-pollution syndrome;

- knowing your risks is essential to reducing them.

A Family Like Yours?

Before we get to the questionnaire, let me introduce you to a mother, perhaps much like you, or someone you know. I met this woman and her family at our local library.

After discussing books, including this one, she asked if she could read it. It was still in process so I sent her sections to read, inviting her feedback.

Here's an excerpt of what she wrote:

> Sorry that it's taken me so long to get back to you about the second chapter. I think that I had some fear around what I might learn – after all the evidence in part one. So there was some resistance for me to overcome before I could read it properly!
>
> I was definitely intimidated by the checklists in Strategy 2. I have so many of the symptoms.
>
> I think also, that it might be useful to suggest to the reader that they do a cost/benefit analysis ie. what is the potential long term risk of EMR exposure vs. what is the potential loss that they will incur by restricting their EMR exposure.
>
> They will probably find that many of the lifestyle changes required to restrict EMR are not life-threatening--but are actually life enhancing.

As you'll see in the questionnaire that follows, there's a surprisingly long list of symptoms and conditions that may be linked to EMR exposure; this is because every cell and system in the body is adversely affected. It can be challenging to figure out whether EMR is a factor in an individual's case. More about this in Strategies 3 and 4.

The Radiation Rescue Questionnaire©

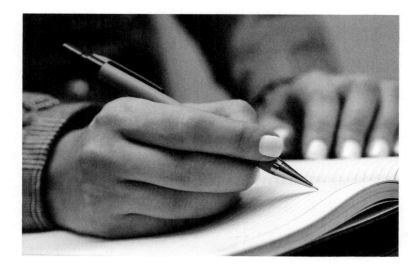

The information contained within the questionnaire does not provide medical advice and is not intended for use in medical diagnosis or treatment.

In the case of any disease, you should always consult your health care practitioner.

You'll notice this survey is not scored; that's because there is no way at this time to weight the effects of the various exposures. While the power of your mobile phone makes a big difference so does the usage.

For example, **Professor Hardell's early research indicated that 500 minutes a month (less than 30 minutes a day) of cell phone use significantly increases brain cancer risk – as much as 140%.**

Other studies show up to a 300 per cent increase when using the cell phone between 500 and 1000 minutes per month.

Source: Wire Technology Research, Second State of the Science Colloquium Book; January 2001 Journal of the American Medical Association; Early Hardell studies.

We need to find out how much the risk increases when combined with exposure to wireless radiation, cordless phones and/or overhead power lines. As Professor Johansson cautions, we are part of that experiment.

I created this questionnaire by extensive research and input from many experts and documents compiled by others. I had the editing assistance of Dr. Heather McKinney. In 2007, she and I reserved editorial control. If you wish to use it in any form, please contact me via the website: www.radiationrescue.org.

Can you connect the dots?

This is one of the objectives of our risk reduction plan.

Is the radiation from your cell phone, and/or cordless phone, one of the reasons you can't sleep? Maybe it's not just the worry.

Is the wireless router in your home, and in their schools, why your children need new glasses again, and are having trouble concentrating?

Is the PDA – always powered on – in your husband's pocket the reason he is having cardiac symptoms? Maybe it's not just the stress.

As you answer the questions in Sections III and IV, you will see your exposures. Then you may see a connection with the Symptoms and Conditions that you answered in I and II. Reduce your exposures with our action plan and see if your symptoms improve.

Section I – Symptoms: Please check those that may affect you when you are exposed to wired, and/or wireless, devices.

- ☐ Abdominal pain
- ☐ Aggressive moods
- ☐ Anxiety or depressive disorders
- ☐ Dry or painful eyes
- ☐ Erratic blood pressure
- ☐ Excessive sweating at night
- ☐ Fatigue
- ☐ Hair loss
- ☐ Headaches
- ☐ Heart palpitations/irregular heartbeat
- ☐ Inability to focus
- ☐ Irritability
- ☐ Libido disturbances
- ☐ Light-headedness/dizziness
- ☐ Loss of appetite
- ☐ Memory loss
- ☐ Menstrual flooding/irregularities
- ☐ Metallic taste in mouth
- ☐ Nausea
- ☐ Nightmares
- ☐ Pain/discomfort in the heart area
- ☐ Pain in the head, neck, shoulders, back
- ☐ Panic attacks
- ☐ Ringing of the ears
- ☐ Sensitivity to noise and/or light
- ☐ Sleep problems
- ☐ Skin rashes/bumps/dryness
- ☐ Tingling and/or numbness
  – in the head, hands and/or feet
- ☐ Vision problems

Section II – Conditions: Please check the items that apply only to your personal health history.

- ☐ Adrenal overload
- ☐ Allergies
- ☐ ALS/Motor Neuron Diseases
- ☐ Alzheimer's Disease
- ☐ Autism Spectrum Disorder
- ☐ Brain aneurism
- ☐ Cancer
  - ☐ Eye
  - ☐ Ear
  - ☐ Brain (adult or child)
  - ☐ Breast
  - ☐ Testicular
  - ☐ Other
- ☐ Leukemia (adult or child)
- ☐ Lymphoma
- ☐ Candidiasis
- ☐ Cataracts
- ☐ Cardiovascular disease
  - ☐ arrhythmia
  - ☐ heart attack
  - ☐ hypertension
  - ☐ stroke
  - ☐ tachycardia
  - ☐ TIA (Transient Ischemic Attack)
- ☐ Chronic Fatigue Syndrome

- ☐ Cold or flu (persistent)
- ☐ Dementia
- ☐ Fibromyalgia
- ☐ Food sensitivities
- ☐ Heavy metal toxicity
- ☐ Infertility
- ☐ Insomnia
- ☐ Irritable Bowel Syndrome
- ☐ Leaky gut syndrome
- ☐ Learning Disorder
  - ☐ ADD
  - ☐ ADHD
- ☐ Lupus
- ☐ Lyme Disease
- ☐ Migraine, or other severe headaches
- ☐ Miscarriage
- ☐ Multiple Chemical Sensitivities (MCS)
- ☐ Multiple-sclerosis
- ☐ Parkinson's Disease
- ☐ Sleep disorder
- ☐ Systemic infection
- ☐ Thyroid gland disorders

Do any of these conditions feel worse when you are exposed to wired, and/or wireless, devices?

☐ No ☐ Yes ☐ I don't know

Section III – Sources of EMR Exposure – Wireless Devices: Please check 'Yes', or 'I don't know' in the columns, as appropriate. Leave an item blank to signify 'No'.

	Yes	I don't know.
Do you regularly use a cell/mobile phone?	☐	
If Yes:		
Less than 4 minutes daily?	☐	
More than 30 minutes daily?	☐	
More than 60 minutes daily?	☐	
In your car?	☐	
For ten years or more?	☐	
Do you experience Symptoms with use?	☐	☐
If No:		
Do you experience any Symptoms around cell/mobile phones?	☐	☐
Do you use a wireless in-your-ear cell phone?	☐	
Do you use a hand-held PDA (personal digital assistant)	☐	
If Yes:		
Less than 4 minutes daily?	☐	
More than 30 minutes daily?	☐	
More than 60 minutes daily?	☐	
In your car?	☐	
For ten years or more?	☐	
Do you experience Symptoms with use?	☐	☐
If No:		
Do you experience Symptoms when you are around PDA's?	☐	☐

	Yes	I don't know.
Have you ever checked the SAR (radiation absorption level) of your cell phone/PDA?	☐	

Do you...

Have your cell phone and/or PDA powered on at night?	☐	
Use your cell phone and/or PDA as an alarm clock?	☐	
Use a headset or ear piece with your mobile?	☐	

If Yes: Check the type you use

    ☐ Wireless   ☐ Wired

Use a wireless game station, or wireless video box?	☐	
Use a wireless device with Internet access, or that downloads music, movies or other wireless transmitted data?	☐	
Use a portable satellite, or wireless broadband, radio?	☐	
Have a GPS, satellite radio, or wireless system, in your car?	☐	
Drive a commercial vehicle with a satellite/GPS locator?	☐	
Use a personal computer connected to wireless Internet?	☐	

Have wireless Internet access....

a) in your home?	☐	
b) in your workplace, school wireless?	☐	☐
c) in your neighborhood?	☐	☐
d) in your city?	☐	☐

	Yes	**I don't know.**
Live or work near a cell tower, or mast?	☐	☐

If Yes:

	Yes	**I don't know.**
a) Within 100 metres? (110 yards)	☐	☐
b) Within 200 metres? (220 yards)	☐	☐
Work with, or live near, radar devices/systems?	☐	☐
Use an amateur radio, 2-way or CB radio?	☐	
Have a cordless/portable phone?	☐	

If Yes:

	Yes	**I don't know.**
a) In your home/office/school?	☐	
b) In your bedroom?	☐	

c) Your total number of cordless phones, and/or baby monitors is:

1_____   2 _____   3_____   4_____

Are your cordless/portable phones

	Yes	**I don't know.**
900 MHz	☐	☐
2.4 GHz	☐	☐
5.8 GHz	☐	☐
DECT 6.0	☐	☐
Have a wireless SmartMeter installed by your utility company at your home/apartment?	☐	☐
Live near a wireless SmartMeter hub and/or SmartGrid network?	☐	☐
Around wireless "hot spots", or devices, do you experience Symptoms from Section I?	☐	☐

Other exposures:

	Yes	I don't know.
Are you an airplane pilot or flight attendant?	☐	
Do you travel often, and go through security X-ray scanners?	☐	
Are you going through *whole body* X-ray scanners?	☐	☐
Do you work at a supermarket checkout or library near scanners, or go through security X-ray scanners at your workplace?	☐	
Have you had a CT scan?	☐	
Have you had an MRI?	☐	
Have you had medical diagnostic X-rays (chest etc.)	☐	
Have you had dental X-rays?	☐	
Have you had a long-term hospital stay – more than one week?	☐	

Section IV – Sources of EMR Exposure – Electric Devices:

Please check 'Yes', or 'I don't know', as appropriate. Leave an item blank to signify 'No'.

	Yes	I don't know.
Do you...		
Use an electric blanket, and/or heating pad?	☐	
Sleep on a/an:		
a) Electric adjustable bed?	☐	
b) Metal bed frame?	☐	
c) Coiled mattress/box springs?	☐	
d) Electrically-heated mattress or water bed?	☐	
Sleep within 2 metres (2.2 yards) of electric devices, including: a clock, radio, compact fluorescent, or low voltage halogen, lights?	☐	
Sleep within 6 metres (6.5 yards) of an electrical fuse panel?	☐	
Stay in a hotel more than five nights per month?	☐	
Regularly use a hairdryer and/or electric shaver?	☐	
Use a microwave oven?	☐	
Are you often by the front burners of an electric stove while they are operational?	☐	
Are you often near electric heaters or "off-peak" or "overnight" electric storage heaters?	☐	
Do you...		
Live/work/school near overhead power lines?	☐	☐
Live in a densely populated urban area?	☐	

	Yes	I don't know.
Work/live near electrical transformers?	☐	☐
Work/live near a electrical sub-station?	☐	☐
Live/work near an airport?	☐	☐
If Yes:		
a) Within 0-5 km? (0-3 Miles)	☐	☐
b) Within 5-15 km? (3-9 miles)	☐	☐
Work/live in a brightly lit room more than 5 hours daily?	☐	
Work with power tools?	☐	
Work with other electrical, or high frequency, equipment?	☐	
Does your home/work have dimmer switches on any lights?	☐	
Do you have low voltage halogen, tube or compact fluorescent, lights at work and/or at home or school?	☐	
Do you live/work in an area with high radon gas?	☐	☐
Do you drive/ride in a hybrid car (gas/electric), or a car with wireless Internet and other high-tech electronics?	☐	
Do you experience Symptoms from Section I around electric devices?	☐	☐

As you know, when artificial electricity was introduced it was a whole new kind of energy that created many obvious advantages and some great gadgets. Obviously, there's harm if you put your finger in a live socket, but generally, we have come to view electronics as benign; this may explain why many people sleep with a cell phone close by their heads without concern. I'm hoping that by now you are viewing our electrified conveniences in a more cautious light.

You may well be thinking, "Okay, I've got it. What can I do about this problem?" So, let's get on with it.

To begin, we need a quick crash course.

Why do we need to know the EMR basics?

You don't really need to be an expert in the various kinds of radiation to reduce your exposure. However, you want to be sure that you are decreasing, not increasing, your electro-magnetic load. (This is an important reminder for the get-on-with-it types who dive into assembling something without reading the instructions.)

Here's an example of a little knowledge being a less-than-safe thing. I visited a friend who has a few testing meters. I was surprised to see she was standing close to her microwave oven when it was on. I asked gently if she felt this was safe. She said, "It's okay, no problem. I tested it and it's fine at this distance." She was using her Gauss meter, which tests the magnetic field around this plugged in appliance. She didn't, however, test the microwave radiation with the instrument which measures that – the RF meter. Not only did she test the wrong exposure, she missed the most harmful one. More on this in a few pages...

The Electro-magnetic Spectrum

So here's what you need to know.

An electric field is the energy surrounding wiring in the walls, or an electric device, extension/power cord that is plugged in. (Note: there is an electric field around everything that is plugged in, even when it is turned OFF. Surprised?)

A magnetic field is the energy surrounding the same wires or appliances when an electrical current is flowing – for example, the lamp is turned on.

Radio-frequency (RF) radiation – these wireless waves (fields) are also called microwave radiation. Here the frequency is so high that small packets of energy are released from the antenna – as in mobile devices. In the case of a microwave oven, you can cook with these waves.

Electro-magnetic radiation (EMR) – also known as **electro-magnetic fields (EMF)** – is the over arching term for most of the spectrum – see the next page. Technically, EMR/EMF includes everything but the highest frequencies (ionizing radiation – X-rays etc).

The Three Windows

A. Lower Frequencies	B. Higher Frequencies	C. Highest Frequencies
Electricity	**Microwaves/Radio-frequency**	
	Wireless except microwave ovens	Nuclear material
Power lines		The Sun
Transformers	Microwave ovens	Cosmic Rays
Electrical wiring	Fluorescent lights	Gamma Rays
Plug-in appliances	Satellite uplinks	CT Scans
Electric blankets	Cell tower antennas	Medical X-rays
Electric heaters	Wi-Fi, wLAN, Wi-MAX	Dental X-rays
Electric shavers	Cell phones - PDAs	Airport security scanners
Hair dryers	Cordless phones - DECT	Ultraviolet (fluorescent lights)
Power tools	Wireless: devices/games/speakers	
Office equipment	headsets, earpieces	TEST WITH instruments that
Lamps, light fixtures	RF identification tags	measure X and gamma rays,
Dimmer switches	Baby monitors	like a GEIGER COUNTER
Electric clocks	Security systems	or a SCINTILLATION
Power cords	Dimmer switches	COUNTER.
Extension cords	Police and other radar devices	
Power bars	Pagers, Walkie-talkies	
Computers	Radio-frequency sealers	
TVs - Video Display Terminals	Radio AM/FM, CB radios	
Plumbing current	GPS systems	
Electric Fields - TEST WITH	TEST WITH RF METER	
ELECTRIC FIELD METER		
Magnetic Fields - TEST WITH		
GAUSS METER		

As you see, there are three basic kinds of frequencies.

A. Lower Frequencies: (electric and magnetic)
Electric fields are emitted by:

- Household electrical wiring in ceilings, walls and floors; wiring that powers lights and appliances

- Everyday power cords, extension cords, and power bars when plugged into an outlet, even if the appliance is not turned on

- Electric blankets, waterbeds, TVs, computers and all other electronic devices

- All electrical appliances, lamps and lighting

- High voltage power lines

Electric fields are tested by:

- An electric field meter

Magnetic fields are emitted by:

- High voltage power lines
- Electrical wiring errors and current on the electrical grounding system, water and gas pipes
- Electric meter and fuse box, dimmer switches, all power transformers/AC adapters
- Fluorescent and low voltage halogen lighting, alarm clocks
- Heating elements in stoves and ovens when heating
- All appliances (refrigerator, washing machine, furnace, hair dryers, exhaust fans etc...)
- All CRT (cathode ray tube) VDT (video display terminal) televisions and computer monitors (in some cases, LCD displays are a better choice but some still emit hazardous levels of EMR.)
- Automobile engines

Magnetic fields are tested by:

- A magnetic field, or Gauss, meter.

B. Higher Frequencies: (the middle – the wireless – window) Microwaves/Radio-frequency fields are emitted by:

- Baby monitors, wireless security systems, wireless game pads, and microwave ovens
- Cellular tower base stations, cellular phones, hand-held PDAs, all cordless phones, wireless technology

- Wireless computer networks and Internet access routers

- All other wireless communication devices

- Some other sources include: fluorescent lights, PUC (under counter lights), some remote control toys, laptops in wireless mode, and some hydro, gas and water meters

Higher Frequencies are tested by:

- An RF meter.

C. The Highest Frequencies:

The third kind of energy shown on the chart is a powerful force, which can create significant cell damage if there's enough power, proximity and duration. This is why it is now recommended to limit X-ray exposure to medically-urgent situations. Other sources include: radioactive mineral deposits, radon gas, nuclear facilities and fallout, depleted uranium such as some troops deploy in combat, and household smoke detectors that contain americium dioxide.

We are all exposed to cosmic radiation to some degree; it's most significant at high altitudes, or in airplanes. At 36,000 ft. the levels can be hundreds of times higher than on the ground.

The Highest Frequencies are tested by:

- Instruments that measure X and gamma rays, like a Geiger counter or a scintillation counter.

Whether or not these or any other exposures are harmful depends on some significant variables. With each exposure you want to consider these factors.

Six Key Factors:

Evidence of harm – as we have discussed, even electro-magnetic levels far below existing 'safe' standards, not high enough to heat human tissue, cause adverse biological effects.

The evidence? See the first section of this book, or some of the Resources' websites. The Resources are at the end of the book.

Intensity – the power of the specific source: the type and power of your cordless phone – analog or digital – 900 MHz to DECT 6.0; and the range of the cell towers, broadcast antennas, power lines, wireless networks etc.

Proximity – how close you are to the source. Is the cell phone against your ear; the wireless laptop on your lap; the cordless phone base nearby; the cell tower, transformer, electric sub-station, or power lines near your house/school/workplace? Your neighbors' wireless network is exposing your family, but is less harmful than having one in your own home – due to proximity.

Duration/frequency – if you have a high-powered electric heater (intensity) on for ten minutes to take the chill off the room, no big deal. If you sleep beside it, or have it on for hours every day (proximity, duration and frequency) that's more of a concern.

Vulnerability – fetuses, infants, children or teens, with thinner skulls, still-growing brains and more aqueous brain tissue, are at greatest risk. Older people, cancer survivors, and those with compromised immune systems, learning disorders and other medical and neurological conditions, are also vulnerable.

Combination of factors – the more of these factors that are present, the greater the danger, as you would presume. A baby sleeping near a wireless monitor, an electric outlet, and a cordless phone, in a home with a wireless security system and wireless Internet is surrounded by multiple, accumulating exposures.

Before I knew about all this, I gave my 85 year-old mother a heating pad to improve her circulation. She began sleeping with it held against her tummy. Shortly afterwards she began to experience uterine bleeding and was taken to hospital to be checked out.

Fortunately, this was about the time I found out about EMR, and that it could cause internal bleeding. My mother's doctor dismissed quickly this information, but we removed the heating pad anyway, and the bleeding stopped within 24 hours. (As with our daughter's metal canopy bed frame, I couldn't bring myself to give the heating pad to anyone else.) All factors were present: the EMR intensity of the heating pad, the proximity of having it next to her body, the duration and frequency of using it all night every night, and her vulnerability from age and health conditions.

Another example: a fragile premature infant in an incubator, hooked up to all kinds of life-saving electrodes and monitoring equipment. Adding to the infant's exposure is the hospital's electro-magnetic load – fluorescent lighting, wireless systems etc. The hospital may even have a large cell antenna on its roof.

Before we go to Strategy 3 – Safer Solutions, here's our library mum:

> Made a few changes since reading Strategy 2 last night. Thought about how I also use my new multi-task cell phone to listen to music, and for a bedside alarm. Turned it off for the night, as well as both computers which were humming away. Put 'get battery alarm clock' on my to do list. Am contemplating getting rid of this all-in-one phone and scaling back to the simpler cell phone.
>
> And I am feeling like we need to get outside more. Unplug.

2 Minute Quick Read Summary

Strategy 3. Safer Solutions

TO REDUCE THE RISKS of electro-pollution is our goal. In Strategy 3 you learn about the emitting devices/exposures and what to do about them. They are grouped into wireless and wired.

Includes the safer use of:

- cell phones
- hand-held PDAs
- headsets
- cordless phones
- Internet access
- laptops
- computer screens
- baby monitors
- video gaming
- microwave ovens
- fluorescent lights
- diagnostic X-rays
- plasma TVs
- electric/hybrid cars

You might know a lot about cell phones but the health benefits of replacing your cordless phones with corded landlines may surprise you. May I suggest you try it and see if your sleep improves.

Look here for our definitive guide to headsets. Guess what? Wireless ones are *not* the safest, our technical team tells us.

Learn about Smart Meters and wireless radiation in schools, and how to make sure our children are healthy. Read about Wi-Fi in transportation and why we don't want pilots exposed to any more radiation, even if it's convenient for us to be online while flying.

You don't need to tackle all devices/exposures at once. Every reduction lowers long-term risk, and there are short-term benefits.

See Strategy 3 for more details.

Strategy 3. Safer Solutions

Here's all the information you need to know about the EMR-emitting devices in your home, office, school ...

In this section we look at the specific devices – cell phones, headsets, cordless phones, baby monitors, Internet access etc. – and hear from some of world's leading technical experts including: Alasdair Philips, Rob Metzinger, Larry Gust and Stan Hartman, Katharina Gustavs and Chris Anderson. This is what we, the consumers, have needed to know.

This is probably more than you *want* to know about many of your favorite things. I'm hoping that you won't go from techno-crazed to techno-phobic – there is a healthy balance in the middle way. The technical truth about these devices has been a four year discovery for me; I have had time to go through my stages of denial, anger, action and adjustment.

I don't want you to feel so swamped with these details that you abandon this rescue project altogether. If you find yourself feeling exasperated – "Oh no, not my hair dryer" – please take a break and come back to this another day.

Over time, if you can just tackle a few of the 'biggies' – such as the cordless phone – you have done a lot to safeguard your family.

How can you decide whether devices are safe or not?

Let's use the analogy of sun tanning. You know that while we need some exposure to the sun (evidence of benefit), too much can be hazardous (evidence of harm). It follows that caution is advised when being outside in the mid-day sun (intensity), or using sun lamps or tanning beds (intensity and proximity).

According to our experts, if you are using a powerful device (intensity), on a regular basis (duration), wearing it on your body, sleeping near it, or holding it in your lap – or against your head (proximity), you are at risk. You can see why there's so much concern about cordless and mobile phones.

Mobile Alert: Even Higher-Powered Tech Toys on the Electronic Horizon

An eye of awareness can wake us up when we see advertisements touting the latest high-tech toys: a compact wireless "netbook", a formidable DECT 6.0 cordless phone station to control all the functions in your home, a pink pendant cell phone that nestles in your

cleavage, a wireless exercise pad for "Wi-Fi fitness", and mobile online banking services – right from your cell phone.

Here's one to jolt your alert button: we are promised a 4G multi-function mobile that will "be like your very own butler in the palm of your hand. It'll do everything but tuck you in at night."

Get your radiation-testing meter ready.

The Key Question: Does it work without wires?

Many people are concerned about living near power lines, or electric sub-stations. This risk is validated by extensive research. However, we are just learning of the risk of the radiation from cell towers.

Somehow these massive structures do seem menacing (of course, that's why they are often concealed in metal church crosses, or disguised as palm trees). Yet, the digital cordless phone sitting on your kitchen counter looks so benign. The new digital baby monitor seems to be essential for safety-minded parents. And in this digital age it seems an educational advantage to start our children young in becoming at home with computers – usually with wireless connection to the Internet.

For something to communicate without wires, it uses some form of radiation to send and/or receive data through the air. Most of these waves travel easily through cement walls. This means they are also going through the skull, and the rest of the body.

The Key to the Safer Solutions

Stan Hartman, an environmental health consultant, offers us key advice:

> The most important thing for people to keep in mind when trying to reduce electro-smog is, first of all, to replace all wireless technology (except infrared remote controls for TVs and other things) with wired alternatives.
>
> Get rid of all bluetooth devices, and replace other wireless gear like cordless speakers, headphones, keyboards, mice, etc.

If the data transmission is going through a hard-wired cable, a plugged-in phone line, or a fiber optics system, then it does not present that kind of exposure. These differences form the basis of the safer solutions.

When you have this awareness these decisions seem to arise instinctively. And wiser choices become obvious. You can decide, for example, how to set up your online banking.

If you're using a device that has a thin LCD screen (vs. the larger cathode ray terminal) and hard-wired Internet access (instead of wireless), you can enjoy that convenience with much less risk than using your cell phone or PDA.

The Sources and Recommendations

In this section we'll look at exposures from various sources, explain the experts' concerns about them, and suggest safer solutions.

It is important to know the difference between making something safer, and making it safe. For example, when you add a filter to a plain cigarette does it make it safe? If it is a low tar cigarette does it make it safe? If you only breathe in second hand smoke, does it make it safe?

As you read through this section, you will get an idea of the exposures you want to reduce. At the end of this strategy there is a preliminary Action Plan to help you prioritize; you'll find a more detailed version at the end of Strategy 4.

We are going to start with the devices from the higher frequencies – the middle of the EMR Spectrum.

Microwave Ovens

The Concern: Larry Gust, an electrical engineer, tells us why that handy appliance is not as harmless as it looks.

(LG) "All microwave ovens leak RF radiation (radio-frequency, microwaves) when they are in use. This radiation covers a surprisingly wide area – as much as 3 to 30 feet, and in older models up to 60 feet. Most people think that microwave ovens do not have any negative health consequences.

After all, if they did the government would not allow this product on the market. Think again.

The Soviet Union conducted extensive microwave research after finding German microwave ovens and research data at the end of WWII. Unhampered by capitalistic trade associations, Russian research has been more extensive than that in the US. This article summarizes early Russian and other more recent research.

Microwave ovens use electromagnetic energy that vibrates 2.4 billion times per second. This energy acts on the molecules in food, particularly water molecules, causing them to vibrate rapidly. This rapid movement generates friction and thus heat. Vibration is so violent that molecules are often torn apart or distorted, thereby changing the chemical makeup of the food. Additionally, this appliance leaks microwaves into the environment around it.

Studies of the thousands of Russian workers exposed to radar microwaves in the 1950's showed health effects so severe that the Russian microwave oven leakage limit was set at 1,000 times less than the US government leakage limit.

In 1976, microwave ovens were banned in the Soviet Union after researchers discovered that these devices caused a breakdown in the human (and animal) energy field. They also found degeneration of cell membranes and electrical nerve impulses in the brain, disruption of hormone production, and disturbance in various brain waves, leading to memory and concentration loss, slowing of intellectual process and interrupted sleep. Microwave ovens were allowed after 1987 when, under Perestroika, business interests pressured Gorbachev into changing the regulations that did not fit in with free-trade practices in the West."

Microwaving baby milk is not recommended. In the December 9, 1989 issue of the British medical journal, *Lancet*, Dr. Lita Lee reported that heating formula in a microwave oven converted some of the amino acids in it into synthetic forms that are not biologically active. One was converted to a toxic form.

Dr. Lee is concerned:

> It's bad enough that many babies are not nursed, but now they are given fake milk (baby formula) made even more toxic via microwaving.

Microwave Ovens – Safer Solutions:

Rob Metzinger (RM): "Replace microwave ovens with safer appliances and methods."

- If you absolutely must have a microwave oven get a smaller, lowered powered one and stand at least 15 feet away – even farther, to be on the safe side – when it is in use.

- Avoid heating baby formula in a microwave, and keep infants and children far away when it is on.

- Better alternatives: keep a small pot or pan with a lid for quick heating/reheating of food and liquids. Avoid non-stick coated pans. (As soon as they are the least bit scratched, you can ingest the toxic little flakes.) At work, heating your lunchtime leftovers in a toaster oven, or on a hot plate with the small pan and lid, takes a couple of minutes longer, but is a safer solution, the experts advise us.

- If you need something defrosted, take it out of the freezer a night or two beforehand and defrost in the fridge.

Cordless Phones

The Concern: You may have known about the hazards of microwave ovens, and been wary of cell phones, but did you know about the health hazards of cordless phones? These conveniences emit high levels of radiation, particularly the newer ones, even when not in use.

Did you know that multiple cordless phone sets that come with a base station, and a charger for each handset, emit two kinds of radiation? The charger sends out harmful magnetic fields within 1 to 3 ft. (The emission of magnetic fields applies to all phones, cordless or not, that come with a cube-style adapter.)

The main base station of a cordless phone, however, is the more dangerous, as the antenna radiates microwaves continually for hundreds of feet/meters. Microwave radiation is also coming from the handset antenna. This is why all the experts urge us not to allow young children near cordless phones. Replacing them should be a key factor in your Action Plan.

From a January 2006 report by the German Federal Agency For Radiation Protection, *The Radiation Source at Home – cordless phones radiate unnecessarily:*

> A cordless phone (of DECT standard – 5.8 GHz or DECT 6.0) is often the strongest source of high frequency electromagnetic radiation in a private home. To renounce your cordless phone as a precautionary measure will contribute to minimizing your family's radiation exposure.

DIGITAL CORDLESS PHONES – ALWAYS RADIATING

 Beginning in 2008, phones of the DECT 6.0 generation started flooding the US market. DECT is the abbreviation for Digital Enhanced Cordless Telecommunication technology. In the last decade, only Europeans used this technology and were confronted with its headaches.

The 2.4 GHz band has been used by the majority of cordless phones in the last five years. However, this band has become crowded with devices such as microwave ovens, wireless area networks (WLAN), Bluetooth, cordless phones and remote control devices. This has led to interference and performance issues so the manufacturers moved to the 5.8 GHz frequency band and then to DECT 6.0 technology.

The problem with the DECT phones is that the base station is permanently sending (radiating) 24 hours a day, no matter if the system is in use or not. Indoor environmental consultants have rallied against their use for decades. There were so many outcries that it had an impact. Major European manufacturers now offer environmentally safer versions, with sleep mode or reduced output in standby mode.

Case Study

Clients are concerned about the installation of a new cellular base station to be erected on the roof of a recreation center across the street from their house and asked to have their home assessed prior to the installation.

Outside
9 μW/m^2

Master bedroom
13,500 μW/m^2

Family room
50 μW/m^2

Office with phone
33,800 μW/m^2

Bedroom 2
5,400 μW/m^2

Bedroom 3
680 μW/m^2

Living room
140 μW/m^2

Entry

(Please don't be scared off by the symbol μW/m2 in this picture, these are the same measures as our RF table.)

RF Exposure from One 2.4 GHz Cordless Phone in a House (these levels are *only* from the cordless phone)

When Peter Sierck sent me this paper on cordless phones, with the RF levels you see in this graphic, I couldn't quite believe that these readings were coming from *one* cordless phone.

He assured me that, "yes, these RF levels are from one 2.4 GHz cordless phone in the house, no wireless, cordless or other RF sources."

Can you just imagine the levels with a few 5.8 or DECT 6.0 phones in a similar house equipped with wireless Internet?

Another widely respected technical expert, Alasdair Philips, the director of Powerwatch in the UK, cautions:

> It's likely everyone in a house with a (DECT) digital cordless phone will be constantly exposed to levels of microwave radiation far higher than safe levels.

Dr. Hans Scheiner, the physician in Munich, also warns us about digital phones (virtually all new/recent cordless phones):

> Digital signals are more aggressive than analog. Both are harmful. However, digital signals are more aggressive, and more harmful, because they pulse and have peaks. This is a problem as the body's cells react negatively to the sharp peaks.

I know; all these health hazard alerts about cordless phones were a shock to me too. I invite you to consider this as good news and bypass the stage of remorse at having placed these phones throughout the house, and choose instead to hear this message.

Ready for another story? A good news one? I have a dear friend who moved into a small duplex near the waterfront, several years ago. She was thrilled to have found this 'fixer-upper' with a wide porch where she could sit and watch the waves; until she discovered that those were not the only waves hitting her haven by the sea. Since moving in, for no known reason, she was not sleeping well and her Chronic Fatigue symptoms were worsening daily.

Right across from her, not too far from shore, was a small island sprouting several broadcast antennas. This was around the time of the dawning of my wireless awareness so I shared with her what I was learning. She is a doctor with a keen and curious mind so she delved head first into the data. And soon took action.

My friend hired an EMR assessment consultant to do some testing. He identified what we had both suspected – radio-frequency radiation from the antennas across the water, and the wireless network in her home. She replaced her wireless with an Ethernet cable, and that seemed to help, but not enough. The consultant had also discovered another source that surprised us, but not him.

The person living in the other half of their duplex had a digital cordless phone that was blitzing the whole building, and way past the surrounding garden. (This may seem more credible to you after just seeing Peter Sierck's diagram of the house plan.)

Fortunately, the elderly woman who lived there was open to hearing about this, although she couldn't quite believe it, "My dear, I have had a cordless phone for years. I keep it beside my chair, and my bed, as I am slow getting up."

After she replaced it with a landline – with a sufficiently long cord – she and my friend both reported sleeping much better, and a reduction in several previously unexplained symptoms.

What similar benefits might there be for you and your family? Read on ...

Cordless Phone Models:

There is a huge difference in radiation exposure from lowest to highest power. **Note: One gigahertz (GHz) is equal to 1,000 megahertz (MHz).**

The 900 MHz analog (if you can find one) emits much less radiation than the newest DECT 6.0 model. Evidently, you can walk three blocks with this new mega-powered unit.

This list goes from the least to most harmful according to our technical experts:

900 MHz analog – hard to find, but a good option (only emit RF when in use)

900 MHz digital – avoid the DSS (digital spread spectrum)

2.4 GHz analog – higher levels but the analog signal is less of a concern than the digital

DECT: 2.4 GHz, 5.8 GHz, and 6.0 DECT (1.9 GHz) – all use the same pulsing digital technology and the base station emits RF all the time. Radiation levels vary depending by model and manufacturer. The new DECT 6.0 models can emit extremely high levels – similar to the exposure from cell phones.

The environmental consultant, Katharina Gustavs, advises us that, "some of the DECT cordless phones operate at a higher frequency, which is not detected by all RF meters. In this case, the meter may show nothing, or give a false low level."

Children and Cordless Phones:

Many researchers warn us that children are more vulnerable to the effects of radiation. The child's small size will encourage whole-body exposure, and rapidly dividing cells that are part of the child's growth processes are highly vulnerable to radiation damage.

Do not let a child use a cordless phone; never put the base near children's sleeping or playing area, or use one near them.

Accepting the experts' advice that cordless phones are harmful is most challenging, do you agree? We lived with them for ages. But not with this digital signal and powerful intensity.

Remember, constantly amped-up electronics are not being tested for biological effects. And, there are slews of hyper-smart techies firing on all cylinders to flood the market with wireless gadgets. Unsupervised. Try testing the EMR levels in an electronics store.

Cordless Phones – Safer Solutions:

(RM) "Replace all DECT/digital cordless phones with landline telephones."

Every one of our technical experts, as well as the other contributors, advise replacing cordless phones. This might seem daunting? Tiresome? But as you learn more it will seem like an essential step in your radiation rescue and worth the hassle of stepping over a phone cord now and then.

Radiation Rescue – The Essentials
Corded Landline Phone

- No microwave radiation

- Replacing cordless phones with landlines may be the best reduction you can make in your family's EMR exposure

- Battery-operated ones have minimal electric field and work in power outages

Every expert I spoke with agrees on this. And if you test cordless phones for microwave emissions (yes, the same kind of radiation) you will understand, and dust off your old corded, landline phone, or go out and buy one.

If you want call display, you need a power source; best option is the battery-operated one, you don't even need to plug it into the wall. You can also get good ones with speakerphone function, so you can still multi-task.

An extended coiled cord on the handset enables you to wander even farther while talking on the corded phone. No, it's not as handy as a cordless phone, but there's no comparison in terms of radiation risk.

If having a cordless phone is non-negotiable for you at this time, consider choosing a 900 MHz analog model – if you can still find one.

The advantage is that it doesn't radiate 24/7, just when you are on a call. So it's recommended to keep those discussions brief, "I'll call you back on the landline .."

I went to see if you can still buy the lower-tech 900 MHz and the salesperson looked at me as though I had asked for two soup cans and a string.

Standing beside a stack of bright blue and black boxes of the hottest DECT 6.0, she declared, "Oh, I don't think they make those anymore; no one wants them. People want the latest, the most high-powered."

Cell Phones, PDAs

The Benefit:

In emergencies mobile phones can be a life-saver, literally, and are unlikely to be harmful if use is very brief, limited to urgent calls, and the phone is kept powered off at all other times.

The Concern:

Near Field and Far Field – another bit of crucial information

Cell phones/PDAs emit a laser-like beam of radiation from their antennas, which may be sticking out or embedded in the device. The near field radiates about a foot from the antenna; the most intense plume is within a 7-inch diameter circle around the antenna.

This powerful blast of near field radiation goes into your ear canal and directly to your brain. It also affects your eyes.

The far field, also radiation that causes concern, goes through everything in its path.

The reason you hear that a headset is recommended is that it removes the near field exposure from the area closest to your head and brain. While in a relative sense, it's safer to keep the antenna's near field as far from your brain as possible, as Rob Metzinger explains, the conventional wired and wireless headsets can work against us by increasing the exposure to other sensitive tissues. (There's more about headsets and earpiece phones later.)

Whether or not you're using a headset, when your mobile is clipped to your belt, or carried in your pocket or shoulder bag, you are radiating breasts (remember the pink pendant cell phone?) testicles and other sensitive body parts including organs like liver, kidney and ovaries. There are also concerns about the effect on the blood-producing bone marrow in your hip.

The intensity of radiation lessens with distance, but even the far field is not considered safe, as the information-carrying radio waves are still pulsing through your body for quite a distance.

The more powerful the device, the more intense the near and far field exposures, as you would imagine. Before you grab the latest multi-function mobile, consider testing it with a RF meter. Make sure the phone is transmitting when you test it.

(KG) "The concern with cell phones is not only the very high levels of RF radiation but they also generate very high pulsing magnetic fields, even in standby."

Pregnant Women, Children and Cell Phones

The Concern:

Ronald Herberman, MD, is the first director of the University of Pittsburgh Cancer Institute, a National Cancer Institute (NCI) designated Comprehensive Cancer Center. Dr. Herberman, and his international panel of experts, caution:

> The developing organs of a fetus or child are the most likely to be sensitive to any possible effects of exposure to electromagnetic fields. Do not allow children to use a cell phone, except for emergencies.

Dr. Carrie Hyman, like me, is a concerned parent and advises:

> Parents need to know that our children's developing brains, immune and endocrine systems between the age of conception and mid-twenties (particularly the brain and nervous system) are developing and more vulnerable than an adult's to many toxins, including EMFs. Having a cell phone does not necessarily make your child safer.

There seems to be a consensus among experts that children should not use cell phones, as exposure at a young age is associated with many health problems. Let's hope more governments follow the example of France and other forward-thinking countries.

Alasdair Philips (AP): "Microwaves from mobile phones penetrate the head, and the younger you are, the further into the brain they go, as the skull is thinner and the brain smaller.

Also keep children away from anyone using a mobile phone and don't have one on standby anywhere near a child – on the stroller etc."

Children should not hold any wireless device on their laps, particularly when it is online accessing the Internet, sending or receiving – text messaging etc."

With all of these experts' warnings are you having a hard time taking this in? I know, just about every home is replete with wireless devices. Our children are using them at school, we give them as gifts, they are everywhere.

Another mom who was reading this book commented:

> When I walked into our children's bedrooms, after reading your book, I suddenly realized how many electronic devices were there. Maybe this is why our daughter is not sleeping so well? Why our son is having difficulty focusing? Why they have both had so many colds? And we were going to get rid of our landline as we all had cell phones, even the kids. Read your book just in time.

Many young people may soon wonder, "What's a landline?" PLEASE, I am begging you now, **don't give up your landline**. Yes, it may seem a money-saving move, but at what cost to your wellbeing?

Strategy 3. Safer Solutions

Safe in Standby?

Have you noticed that when people in an audience are asked to turn off their cell phones, most put them on mute/vibrate? This prevents annoying rings, but not the harmful exposure.

When your phone is on standby, it communicates every three to five minutes, at full power, with the nearest base station to ensure it has the best signal. If you are in a poor reception area, the phone may transmit as often as every 30 seconds as it tries to get a better signal. If you are on the move, it will transmit even more frequently.

The various modes of your mobile phone

This list sets out the various settings of a cell phone/PDA, in order of exposure from lowest to highest.

Not emitting radiation:

- battery out – Yes, there is still a tiny bit of energy coming from a mobile that is powered off. Not a concern unless you are electro-sensitive. The only way to reduce the radiation to zero is to remove the phone's battery.

Emitting radiation:

- powered off – be in this safe mode as much as you can.

- charging

- on standby – you can receive calls

- sending receiving text – less harmful if only powered on for a moment to send or receive messages.

- sending and receiving voice, online Internet, downloading movies.

Cell Phones – Less Harmful Solutions

Obviously, the safest solution of all is not to use a cell phone, and try to avoid places where others are using them. Not easy, as you know. When landline phone communication is not possible for you, the following suggestions will at least reduce your exposure.

The Connect Factor

To send data (voice, text and/or images) your mobile has to communicate with the nearest cell tower. The efficiency of this connection is important. The telephone's communication power (TCP) is a measurement of this capacity – how much power it uses to communicate with the cell tower/base station, transferring data *away* from the head which is a good thing. You want a mobile with a high TCP number (see: www.tcodevelopment.com for details.) Now let's look at other factors including your location, frequency of use, how you use the phone, its features, and the radiation emission level, called SAR.

Specific Absorption Rate

SAR is a term used to describe the rate at which tissue absorbs radiation. This is often used as an indication of the level of risk for the radiation-emitting device that is being measured. **As you can imagine, the more 'bells and whistles', the more power, the potential for more harm, we are told.** Choose the most basic phone you can find. As well as taking other precautions, it may be better to choose a device with the lowest SAR. These SAR ratings, however, may not be reliable.

Powerwatch is a leader in this field; the organization's opinion is that SAR ratings are only minimally useful as they are based only on thermal effects. As you may remember, from Know the Evidence, the radiation from cell phones produces harmful biological effects far below thermal levels and existing government standards. For these reasons, relying on a low SAR cell phone could give you a false sense of safety.

(LG) "The way the SAR standard is being subverted to allow more power output has been explained to me that the dimensions of the tissue measured for this test have been altered to have 1/10th the surface area. Therefore the power per unit area is reduced allowing 10 times the power for the same SAR value."

However, it still seems advisable to use a lower SAR cell phone rather than a high one (dealing with relative risk, *not* safety solutions). As the word gets out about the evidence that mobile phones can be harmful, we can expect to see manufacturers' revised ad campaigns: "this low SAR mobile is safe ..." If you want to know the SAR for your mobile, look at this link, where you'll find the Environmental Working Group's ratings of the best and worst phones and PDAs: www.ewg.org/cellphoneradiation/Get-a-Safer-Phone

So our tips begin with choosing a mobile with a high TCP connect factor number, and a low SAR number. Then consider these factors:

Frequency of use

(RM) **"Use cell phones as little as possible. Biological effects occur after 30 seconds**. Only use your cell phone to establish contact, or for conversations lasting a few minutes, as the biological effects are directly related to the duration of exposure.

Your phone communicates at full power when it is connecting to a number, so hold it away from your body when you have finished dialing, until the person answers. This limits the power of the electromagnetic field emitted near your ear and the duration of your exposure. For longer conversations, use a land line with a corded phone, not a cordless phone.

When you are not using your cell phone, turn it completely off (powered off, not on standby) to avoid exposure that is the result of your cell phone transmitting its location through constant signaling.

If you must have your cell phone on, carry it in a purse, backpack or briefcase. Never carry a cell phone that is turned on in any pocket, as the radiation from the phone will couple with your body's natural electro-magnetic field and trigger whole-body adverse biological cascades.

If you must carry your cell phone on you, make sure that the keypad is positioned toward your body and the back (where the antenna is visible, or embedded) is positioned toward the outside so that the transmitted electromagnetic fields move away from you rather than through you.

Avoid having a cell phone near your body at night, under the pillow, or on a bedside table. If you need an alarm consider a much safer alternative such as a battery powered alarm clock."

Want a health-savvy gift? Give your loved one a battery alarm clock.

Type of use

Here are some of the recommendations you need to know: **Never use a cell phone with the antenna within six inches of your body.** As much as possible, use the speakerphone mode so that the antenna can be kept a safer distance away from vulnerable tissues and organs. **Never wear your cell phone in a pocket, or carry it near your heart.**

As a cardiologist, Dr. Sinatra is aware of this concern and reinforces this recommendation, "I would avoid having any wireless device near the heart; this includes a wireless microphone."

Switch sides regularly while communicating on your cell phone to spread out your exposure. It is advisable to use text messaging instead of talking when possible. Hold the phone away from you until the text is sent. Then power it off.

Is your mobile 'amping up'? The bars indicate the strength of the signal in your area; the maximum number of bars is preferable.

It's best to keep your cell phone fully charged, and best not to use it with low battery, and/or in an area of poor reception. And don't talk on the phone when the battery is being charged – that amplifies both the low frequencies (from the electrical connection) and the Information Carrying Radio Waves (the wireless communication).

Charge the phone in an area away from people and pets."

Location of use

Evidently, if you're standing somewhere and turn your cell phone on, and the base station is behind you, the signal goes through you. Yes, through you.

(CA) "When you use your cell phone in an environment where Wi-Fi or Wi-MAX signals are present, the body is subjected to 2 major assaults… these signals tend to couple forming new waveforms, which cause more harm."

We are also advised to refrain from using a cell phone, or other wireless device, in a car, truck, train, boat, airplane or other confined metal perimeter space. When you're inside a metal box your mobile is continually trying to reconnect to the nearest relay antenna, and the signal is trapped inside and bounces around, concentrating the exposure and amplifying the radiation.

And it is not recommended to use your cell phone when moving at high speed, in any mode of transportation, as this automatically increases the mobile's power to a maximum as it makes repeated attempts to connect to a new antenna.

If you must have a phone on in the car, an external roof-mounted antenna will make it less harmful, though dividing your attention between a phone conversation and the road is never a good idea.

 (CA) "Hands free cell phones are reportedly no safer than hand-held ones, as some studies show them being 50% more likely to cause accidents. Moreover, science shows that cell phone radiation impairs reaction time and brain function, so it is clear that the main culprit is not the 'distraction' factor – as claimed by the wireless industry – but the phone radiation which causes impairment and more accidents."

Also, please think about this: other drivers using phones may be suffering from similar impairment, so drive defensively.

Japanese physicists have also found that radiation hot spots often emerge in reflective areas, such as elevators. These researchers say passive radiation exposure is similar to second-hand smoke.

When using a mobile in a building, it is recommended to stand by a door or window and to hold it between you and the outside so less radiation goes through you as the signal blasts to connect with the nearest antenna.

1 Guideline – Limit use of your cell phone.

Have a "no frills" cell phone with speaker function – use it outside of the car, or other confined space. A wired headset is recommended if you cannot use the speakerphone.

- **Keep it turned off as much as you can.**

- Use standby mode only when expecting an urgent call.

- Turn it off – not receiving – when it's charging.

- Use a limited service plan. If you have young people using a mobile device, make sure you check the bill often. Your idea of their having a cell phone to keep them safe, and in touch with you, may not match their communication objectives. The bill will tell the true story. Remember the risk of 500 minutes a month ...

Pagers

Stan Hartman (SH) "If you have to be accessible by phone it's safer to carry a pager. Then when you are paged you can turn on your cell phone to make a quick call, if there is no landline nearby."

Remember this is "safer", reduced risk. Not "safe". Some doctors report people who have pagers have symptoms near where they carry them.

10 Safer Guidelines for Mobile Phones/PDAs

1. Use a landline whenever possible – "May I call you back on my landline?"

2. Use a low-tech, lowest SAR rated phone with a speaker function – avoid the hands free in-the-ear phones.

3. Use on speakerphone, or with a hollow air tube headset.

4. Limit calls, and keep powered off whenever possible.

5. Carry away from your body – at least with the keypad or front of the cell phone facing toward the body, and the back or antenna side facing away from the body.

6. Use outside of a car, train, elevator, airplane or other confined metal space.

7. Use a computer with wired Internet access, with the wireless function disabled, to surf the Internet, watch movies, download music etc. not a mobile.

8. Keep it fully charged (it has to 'amp' up more if the battery is weak, and/or if the reception is poor.)

9. Keep away from your sleep zone, use a battery-operated alarm clock to wake you up. Never sleep with your cell phone powered on. Charge away from humans/pets – not on 'standby' at night.

10. Internet Phones also carry risk – particularly when you're on wireless Internet access.

Wireless Earpiece Phones

The Concern:

One website marketing these all-in-one microphone and speaker wireless ear buds trumpets the advantages: **"Boosting sound and channeling it directly into the ear, reducing interference and noise."** This is *not* all they're channeling.

And, yes, these do keep your hands free for driving, which seems a good idea. However, these devices may be the most harmful of all to your vulnerable eyes and brain.

(RM) **"It is important *not* to have the speaker IN the ear, as with the microphone kind of phone. Magnetic fields go right through the surface so they are active in the brain at close distance."**

Think about the pulsing digital radiation blasting to its host, or base station, and then on to a cell tower every few minutes, even on standby. And where is it also going from its snug position wedged in your ear?

Technology writer Stewart Fist reported from Australia that lab testing of wireless earpiece phones shows **the radiation they give off exceeds current government standards**, and we know about those.

Hands-free While Driving

Oprah Winfrey is on a worthy campaign to make cars a "No Phone Zone" after hearing about a young girl killed by a distracted driver. "A call or text isn't worth taking a life," said Winfrey. "My biggest hope is that it becomes mandatory that no one uses their phone in the car or texts while driving—just as seat belts are mandatory, I'm hoping that this becomes not just law, but second nature for all of us."

Bringing such high-level media attention to this issue is much needed and not always easy to do as the wireless industry is massively powerful.

And Dr. McKinney sent me this – an increasing trend in transportation:

> POLICY: The use of interactive wireless communication devices by employees of The Pennsylvania State University while on University business is prohibited while operating any vehicle.

As we know from the research, wireless radiation can cause cognitive impairment, so this isn't just an issue of multi-tasking. Hands-free is a positive step, but not with a wireless earpiece. The "No Phone Zone", and pulling over to make your brief call, using the speakerphone, are better, our technical experts advise, and could save a life. Maybe yours.

Wireless Earpiece Phones – Safer Solutions:

As noted above, it is highly recommended to use the speakerphone function on a low-tech cell phone – see other headset recommendations on the next few pages.

Cell Phone Headsets

The Concern:

People often ask whether using a headset is safer than holding a mobile phone right to your ear. This seems to make sense. And most experts do recommend using some kind of wired headset, if you cannot use the speakerphone.

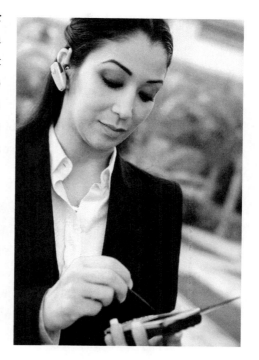

However, **all advise against wireless headsets**. You will see the difference here again between the various levels of reducing exposure, and something being considered relatively safe.

Wireless Headsets

Many experts advise us that most headsets are not safe and that wireless listening devices worn in the ear dramatically increase whole-body radiation exposure and trigger systemic adverse effects.

(RM) "I would not recommend using a wireless headset. Even if they have relatively low power, as compared to the mobile phone, your head's exposure to the additional digital RF-signal will still be above the values recommended in 2008 by IBE (Institute for Bau-Biologie®). It also adds another signal which can increase risk."

Wired Headsets

Unfortunately, this does not seem to be the safe solution, either, as wired headsets are reducing the **near field** only. Yes, the near field is the laser-like intensity closest to your eyes and brain, but the far field is also considered harmful. Larry Gust explains:

(LG) "The wired headset does get the phone away from the head. So the big hammer is removed because you are out of the near field which is 4 times stronger than the far field. However, I have heard commentary that the radio signal follows the wire from the cell phone to the head set."

(RM) "I have concerns about using conventional wired headsets. The high frequencies emitted by the mobile phone will tend to follow the direction of the wire and "lead their way" up to the ear/head.

This is a concentrated emission and can be just as strong as holding the mobile phone directly to the ear. Also, the generation of sound in the earphone speaker produces low frequency AC magnetic fields in the range of 5 Hz to 20,000 Hz.

These fields will easily penetrate the skull since the source is the earphone, directly inside the ear. This is also why using an air tube headset is advantageous."

Headsets – Safer Solutions:

(RM) "Here is a summary of headset options – worst to best:

Worst – Cell phone held up to your ear, using a wireless headset, or a conventional wired headset

Better – The air tube headset is non-conductive thus separating you from the wires and speaker. This makes it better than a conventional wired headset. For best results, ensure the phone is at a distance and you are not in contact with the wire or the phone. Note: adapters for your particular model of phone may be challenging to find.

Best – Using the speaker phone function (away from the body without contacting it) is the safest option but most speaker phones have poor quality sound and do not allow privacy. This is where the air tube headset comes into play.

Safe – Standard landline phone; choose the corded phone, as often as possible. (If you are electro-sensitive, it's best to use the speaker function on the landline.)"

Every expert recommends switching from cell and cordless phones to landlines. You can get high-tech ones with call display, speakerphone function and more...

What did we learn about headsets?

(SH) "An ordinary wired headset will reduce radiation by many magnitudes. The air-tube headset is a kind of speaker that's a lot closer to your body than the speaker if you used the speakerphone function. Using the mobile phone's speakerphone is recommended."

Currently, there's no safe way to use a mobile phone, nor are there any perfect headsets. A problem with the air tube headsets, often marketed to make your cell phone safe, is that none of our experts see them as a completely safe solution. So you are reducing, not eliminating, risk.

And there's a concern that you may talk away on your mobile – cell phone and/or PDA – thinking you are now completely protected. This is the same concern with stick-on chips, discs etc. More on that later.

It seems prudent to limit calls etc. and use as suggested here. When you cannot use the speakerphone then some kind of wired headset is recommended.

I will keep this issue updated on our website. As consumers demand safer solutions, no doubt we will see more 'radiation-reducing' products on the market. Consumer beware.

The key principle that all of our experts agree upon is: if any device is communicating data through the air, wirelessly, use caution.

It's Not Just Children at Risk

When we are exposed to the radiation from mobile phones, and other wireless technology, we must consider the intermediate massive impairment of our micro-circulation, and therewith the oxygen supply of our inner organs and brain, caused by the tendency of our red blood cells to stick together under the influence of radio waves (DR. PETERSOHN 1998, RITTER UND WOLSKI 2005). In addition to this Prof. Kind (Environmental Hygienic Department of Vienna University) found a high increase of heart attacks, strokes, thromboses and embolism in people who live near (cell towers) transmitter masts.   Hans Scheiner, MD

A Summary: the Radiation Rescue Communications Kit

- Corded landline phone – use for all phone calls, whenever possible
- Low-tech cell phone with speakerphone function – for quick, urgent-only calls (see Safer Use Recommendations)
- Wired (air tube?) headset
- Pager – only on at times you must be reachable
- Cable/wired Internet access

A Great Gift

Consider this kit for your family at home, and when your young people leave to set out on their own. Graduation gift?

As you know, many of this young generation are using mobile phones for all their calls and have never had a landline installed where they are living.

A young woman who works in our office is getting married, and we are giving her the first corded landline phone she has ever had since moving away from home.

Of course, it is much more convenient, and less money, not to bother installing a landline and just rely on mobile phone service.

But at what cost to our health? And, there is the consideration that a battery-operated, or not-plugged in, corded phone will keep working during power outages, and when your cell phone is not charged.

Mobile phones have their benefits, as well: great if your car breaks down. Many of our experts told me they keep a fully-charged cell phone – powered off – in the glove compartment of their car.

Video/Wireless Games

The Concern:

Many of these games use wireless technology, both on laptop computers and gaming systems. Much as you may hate the thought of trying to wrest the controller away from the young gamer, there are some concerns you need to know about.

A paper published in 2004 in the medical journal, *Human Reproduction*, reports some devices, when held close to the genitals, raise the temperature in the testicles as much as 3 degrees Celsius. Temperature changes can occur within 15 minutes. Repeated exposure can reduce fertility.

The researchers say that after a few years of daily exposure, the damage may be irreversible, and others report this exposure may be a factor in the increasing rate of testicular cancer in young men.

Computer Game Consoles

(AP) "The transformer which plugs into a power socket emits very high levels of magnetic fields, and should be unplugged when not in use. The hand controls can give off high electric fields."

Other than the considerable health concerns, there's another problem with gaming etc. It keeps our children – of all ages – inside.

Not only is this an unhealthy sedentary lifestyle, they are missing out on being outside. After the rapid-fire explosiveness of the 3-D games, strolling along the beach can seem tediously dull.

Nature, in all its wondrous simplicity, can hardly compete.

Safer Gaming Solutions:

(RM) "Hard-wired is much safer than wireless. Disable the wireless component and replace it with a cable. Encourage your children to use their game systems and laptops on a table or desk, not directly on their laps. And limit use."

(KG) "There are gaming consoles, which will still emit substantial amounts of RF radiation even when the RF antenna from the back is removed and the control devices used are wired! The popular XBOX, for example, will keep radiating as long as it is plugged in."

(AP) "It is advisable to add a grounding wire, and limit use of all video games."

Wireless Internet Access

Even the most humble coffee shop now boasts "free wireless Internet". Hard to believe, I know, but we may see a time when signs declare: "Proud to be wireless free!"

The Concern:

It used to just be cell phones. Now, with our homes, workplaces, schools and whole communities going wireless, the background level of EMR is reaching a very dangerous level.

We have already discussed in detail the mechanism of harm with this wireless radiation.

Alasdair Philips, the electronic engineer who heads Powerwatch, cautions us: "With wireless Internet access the space is filled with pulsing microwave radiation all of the time even when the computers are not in use. (Your techie may not agree.) **We believe that you should avoid using wireless Internet at all costs.**"

Even parks and beaches are going wireless, as you know. Here's a challenge for you: try finding a hotel with wireless-free guest rooms. Almost all are offering wireless – in your room, at the pool and even in the spa. If you operate a hotel or B&B, please consider going back to hard-wired Internet access – you will lead the way when people begin requesting this. And you, and your guests, will probably get a better night's sleep.

Safer Internet Access Solutions

Best Option:

This is a situation where you really need to weigh the risks and benefits, of convenience and your health.

(AP) "It is better to get a cable or ADSL modem/router and run network cables to the rooms where you wish computers to have Internet access. This is not expensive and will avoid irradiating your living and working environment with pulsing microwaves."

(RM) "Replace wireless Internet routers with hard-wired units. Some wireless router models allow the user to shut off the wireless component and convert it to a hard-wired unit. To ensure conversion, test the area around it with a RF detector.

When using a notebook/laptop computer use a hard-wired network connection. Settings to disable the wireless connection are found in Network Settings on a PC, or AirPort on a Mac."

Chris Anderson, an EMR consultant, advises us about wireless Internet:

> As you may know, all computers nowadays are shipped with a default setting that ensures that all wireless networks and systems are turned on as soon as you start your computer. These functions need to be deliberately disabled: go to the Control Panel, click on 'wireless connections', and actually 'disable' the wLAN as well as the 'bluetooth' system.

On a personal note: during my EMR reduction frenzy, I replaced our wireless router with the hard-wired kind. Well, the phone company only had wireless ones, but the techie assured me that there would be no RF/microwave radiation if it wasn't being used wirelessly. Guess what? I had been sitting here at the computer for long hours wondering why I was getting headaches, (of course, there are always other good reasons – eye strain etc).

I decided to test the hard-wired router with a RF (radio-frequency) meter. Even though I had disabled the computer's wireless settings, there were really high RF radiation levels coming from the router. Not good. Evidently, you have to go online to modify the router's settings. Now they tell me!

Another Hard-wired Option:

Networking your Ethernet and your home's power lines

If you cannot use the recommended cable hook-up – wired Internet access – you might consider this new set up where you access the Internet through electrical outlets in the wall. This is not inexpensive, but safer than having all the wireless radiation going through your house, and neighborhood.

(SH) "This is not as good as an ordinary wired modem using Ethernet cable, but way better than Wi-Fi, because the signal is going through the wiring, not through the air. Even if there is some radiation leakage from the wiring, it will be much, much weaker than the exposure from Wi-Fi."

(CA) "This option is NOT the best solution as some RF radiation will spew forth from the entire electrical system."

(RM) "This solution may be a bit dicey because of the dirty electricity issue, which is a bit of an unknown at this point."

Network using powerlines in your home

images courtesy of devolo AG (www.devolo.de)

Another Internet Access Option:

Have at least one computer hard-wired. If you have someone in your house who insists on using a wireless computer in another room, turn on the router for that period of time, then shut it off afterwards. **And make sure a wireless router is turned off at night**. A power bar may be helpful. You could even use one with a timer.

This safer solutions list is from an organization that I regard as the world's leading experts in this field.

How can I protect myself from wireless radiation?

The following tips help to avoid or reduce your personal radiation exposure to wireless networks:

- Always prefer wired data transmission systems to wireless networks (even though you may have to run some wire), especially in residences, schools, and preschools.

- If at all, wireless networks should be run at the lowest possible power output actually required to get the work done (which usually can be set in the software).

- Have access points only transmit for the short period of time required to transfer data, otherwise keep it always turned off, especially during the night. Simply turn the switch at the wireless device off or, better yet, unplug it.

- Preferably, keep transmitting antennas a large distance (>10m or 32.5 ft) away from areas of frequent human use.

- Transmitting antennas should not be installed in the rooms they service but rather in hallways, attics or less used rooms farther away.

- Also keep your neighbor in mind!

- Strategically place access point antennas in such a way as to minimize the radiation exposure in areas of frequent human use. Never connect sector antennas with high antenna gains (and their increased directivity) to access points and never point them towards areas of frequent human use.

- Laptop or PC: Keep your distance from the wireless card; if at any time larger amounts of data are transferred, leave the area. Always turn off the wireless card with a separate switch or disable it in the control panel (PC) or at the task bar (Mac) when not in use.

Perhaps rooms or walls could be specifically shielded if the wireless radiation comes from outside or a neighbor; though it is imperative to have a RF radiation survey conducted prior to any shielding project.

With an external source any solid masonry wall or concrete ceiling reduces RF levels by about 50-80 %, wood frame wall constructions, however, provide hardly any reduction.

One can also cover the wireless device with shielding cloth at night or to reduce the emission level.

W. Maes, F. Mehlis: Wireless Network. A Flyer by the Building Biology Association (VB), 2009. Used with permission. (www.verband-baubiologie.de)

Wireless Systems in Schools

As the principals of my children's schools will tell you, I am a "mother warrior" on this issue.

Another concerned parent, director of a large information technology company, used this analogy:

> If someone put a glass of drinking water in front of you and said we think it's OK to drink and it meets current government standards but there is a substance in it that some credible scientists say may be carcinogenic, would you give your child a glass of that water day after day?

> The scientists and organizations in Europe that are taking positions and actions against Wi-Fi are, in my opinion, highly credible.

> There is no conspiracy here; our governments and institutions have simply not kept pace with the rapid roll out of new technology. Anyone who spends time educating themselves would err on the side of caution.

Anyone who says 'I am not convinced there is a problem with wireless technology' and turns a blind eye is being imprudent. By the time they are convinced, the damage will have been done.

This issue is a dilemma for schools. On the one hand, they're told that information technology gives students an essential educational edge. There's also pressure to go wireless since it's cheaper to install than hard wired systems. On the other hand, what's true of cell phone radiation is equally true of wireless Internet: children are more vulnerable to the biological damage.

The Concern:

Dr. Martin Blank is taking the lead in alerting communities:

> There is enough evidence of a plausible mechanism to link EMF exposure to increased risk of cancer, and therefore of a need to limit exposure, especially of children.

> (Radio-frequency) RF in any form – cell tower radiation, Wi-Fi networks, cell phones etc. – is potentially bad, especially if one is exposed for extended periods (e.g., asleep in bed at home, seated at a desk in school).

Just when I thought I'd heard all the bad news, I read again that epilepsy can be one of the associated EMR conditions, including adult onset. One young man told me about his first seizure – on a transatlantic flight that had Wi-Fi. Maybe no connection, of course, but it is constantly baffling to me why we take such risks with people's health. Need more research here but please consider EMR caution with anyone who has epilepsy, including wireless exposures and even electric heating pads.

Many other eminent scientists including Dr. Gerd Oberfeld and Professor Johansson also have written about the urgent need to remove wireless Internet from schools. They cite the evidence in Strategy 1.

Dr. Magda Havas, Associate Professor, Trent University, sent an open letter to Canadian parents, teachers and school boards in May 2009:

> I am a scientist who does research on the health effects of electromagnetic radiation and I am becoming increasingly concerned that schools are installing Wi-Fi networks and are making their school grounds available for cell phone antennas.
>
> You will be told by both the federal government (Health Canada and Industry Canada) as well as by the Wi-Fi provider that this technology is safe provided that exposures to radio-frequency radiation remain below federal standards. This information is outdated and incorrect based on the growing number of scientific publications that are reporting adverse health and biological effects below our Safety Code 6 standards (see www.bioiniative.org) and the growing number of scientific and medical organizations that are asking for stricter standards to be enforced. For these reasons, it is irresponsible to introduce Wi-Fi microwave radiation into a school environment.

Finally, someone is monitoring this! Dr. Havas has taken a proactive step – much needed – and developed a questionnaire to monitor a child's health in a Wi-Fi school. Ideally, this would be used *before* and after Wi-Fi is installed to track potential symptoms that may, or may not, be related. And this process will increase medical awareness of potential symptoms.

Dr. Sarah Starkey, a UK neuroscientist, set up a website out of concern about the rapid spread of wireless technologies in schools. She has studied the mechanisms underlying learning and memory, circadian rhythms (like our sleep/wake cycles) epilepsy and depression.

According to research on www.wifiinschools.org.uk many of the health risks may only become apparent after years of exposure. Some students and staff could be susceptible to more immediate effects, such as symptoms of electro-hypersensitivity. There are studies that suggest that people with epilepsy have an increased chance of seizures when they're exposed to cell phone signals.

Our international advisory board, Doctors for Safer Schools, is asking legitimate questions about wireless radiation in schools, and requesting accurate answers. We acknowledge we are all part of this biological experiment, as Dr. Salford has warned; however, we must consider our children. How much more evidence do we need before taking protective action? More details at: www.doctorsforsaferschools.org

Wireless Networks, Immune Systems and Viruses

Do you remember that Dr. Scheiner, and other medical experts, have reported wireless radiation suppresses the immune system? With the current spread of the H1N1 virus, and its threat to schools, wouldn't you think that school principals would be more than keen to go back to hard-wired Internet connections and reduce all other exposure levels?

These precautionary steps also make sense in other public spaces, including confined ones like trains, buses and airplanes. Also, you'll read later on what one of our scientists, an immunologist, has to say about wireless radiation and the immune system, and what he recommends if you have to have a flu vaccine (to keep you from skipping ahead, let me tell you here: he suggests the nasal mist, that is mercury-free, instead of the injectable vaccine.)

Educational edge – or irony?

A school principal has made a pitch to the school Board to purchase a wireless Internet network to enhance his students' academic performance. He wants to give them every high-tech advantage. He has read credible research of the many educational benefits of computer technology: better test scores, better learning, better focusing. With the wireless Internet network, and a wireless laptop for each child, he is confident these children will have the leading edge.

 One of the moms is alarmed that her children seem to be even more hyperactive – alternating with fatigue, and occasionally not sleeping well. Sharing her concern with other moms, she discovers their children are also having trouble concentrating; some are experiencing symptoms like headaches, dizziness, nausea, diminishing eyesight, tingling in the hands and impaired immune systems. Two are having difficulty recovering from mononucleosis and Lyme disease.

One parent remarks there were never this many allergies when she was in school. Some test scores are dropping. And there seem to be more 'problem children' who simply can't sit still and focus on their work. These mothers turn their formidable energies toward researching the possible causes – and solutions.

Decrease in Memory, Attention and Ability to Learn?

Electro-magnetic radiation can alter the electrical activity in the brain – with unknown effects on the still-developing brains of children and teens.

As we have seen, scientific studies also show a decrease in cognitive abilities such as memory, attention and decision-making.

Does it makes sense to radiate an educational environment when this exposure has been shown to damage our children, including their ability to sit still, and to learn?

(AP) "School libraries and IT facilities usually have wireless local area networked (wLAN) computers. These can give a high background level of microwaves to which teachers and pupils will be exposed for most of the day.

We are against every pupil having a wireless enabled computer to do his or her school work.

This is because 20 or more computers, with wireless access, fill the classroom with several volts per metre of pulsing microwave radiation electrosmog. Electrically sensitive children will react very badly to this exposure, which is associated with memory and concentration problems and increased aggressive behaviour."

(AP) "**Laptops wired by Ethernet using standard cables are fine.** The pupils can use their laptops on their own for most work and plug in a network cable when they need to access files on the school server computer or on the Internet. Infrared data connections are also believed to be safe."

(AP) "Interactive whiteboards, used to display computer and video images in the classroom also use microwave technology. The whiteboard display (using back or front projection) should be connected by wire to the teacher's controller PC and will not then be a problem.

However, some are now being sold with built-in wireless networks to connect to the teacher's PC and to wireless connected interactive pen displays that can be moved around the classroom and operated by pupils.

These wireless options will increase the ambient level of electrosmog in the classroom."

Wireless Internet in Schools – Safer Solutions:

The obvious solution is to remove the wireless network and go back to the hard-wired system. Dr. Starkey advises parents to take a stand on wireless in their children's classrooms:

> Schools will only use wireless computer networks if the parents want this for their children. Obviously it is not desirable for a few children to be isolated, or to miss out in their education.

> But if parents en masse decide together that their children will only use wired technologies then schools will need to revise their communications technology provision.

How about the safest option – fiber optics?

Visit our website: www.radiationrescue.org for more information on this important issue: the wellbeing of our children *and* teachers and staff working in Wi-Fi schools.

Reducing your child's EMR exposure

- Minimise the time your children play computer games.

- Monitor the type of games they play.

- Keep children at least a metre (3.25 feet) away from working electrical appliances in the kitchen.

- Make sure your child sits at least a metre (3.25 feet) away from the front of a TV screen while watching.

- Position the television set so children cannot spend time to the side or back of it.

- Make sure transformers are kept away from chairs, beds and anywhere a child sits and plays regularly.

- Consider your use of battery-operated equipment. Use rechargeable batteries where possible and dispose of them as toxic waste.

- Position your child's bed away from cupboards containing electric equipment, meters, heaters and the like.

- Make sure all music/entertainment players are plugged in with a grounded cord.

- Make sure your child sits well away from the transmitting unit of a cordless phone system.

- Make sure desk and bedside table lamps are grounded.

- Check your garden for EMR sources and build play areas where field levels are low.

- Make sure your child sits in seats that are not exposed to high EMR in public transport.

- Check your child's nursery and school for sources of EMR.

- Monitor your child's health, behaviour and achievement levels and check school EMR exposure if these deteriorate.

Check whether your child's school has a wireless system or interactive whiteboards. Measure the EMR in the classroom to see if it is at an acceptable level.   (Source: Powerwatch)

Fluorescent Lights

Most people working in offices with overhead fluorescents, whether they are buzzing or not, report eyestrain, fatigue and headaches. The recent promotion of compact fluorescent lights for their energy efficiency causes the scientific community concern. There are two problems with the compact fluorescent lights – one EMR assessment technician calls the CFL "chronic fatigue lights" for their negative impact on our energy. The second problem is they feed what is called dirty electricity back into the electrical system.

Dr. Magda Havas (MH): "Don't use CFL bulbs. These energy efficient compact fluorescent lights generate radio-frequency radiation, ultraviolet radiation, and dirty electricity. Dirty electricity has been shown to adversely affect human health. A recent study of cancer clusters in a school in California associated the increased risk of cancer among teachers to dirty electricity. **CFLs contain mercury – a known neurotoxin** – which can be dangerous once it is released into the environment through breakage or in landfills. With thousands of bulbs sold around the country and inadequate disposal facilities we are setting ourselves up for a mercury time bomb. Compact fluorescent lights are making some people ill, including those who suffer from migraines, epilepsy, skin problems and electrical sensitivity."

Many environmental groups, and governments, are advocating a ban on incandescent lights and mandating the use of CFLs. When you read the science it seems evident we need to find safer ways to cut our energy costs and consumption.

(AP) "Many schools (and workplaces) use fluorescent lighting. The flicker can trigger electrical hypersensitivity and increase antisocial behaviour. If your child develops headaches and/or eye strain, check the school classroom lighting."

Fluorescent Lights – Safer Solutions:

(AP) "Ensure lights are full-spectrum – not fluorescent – as it has been found that people are much healthier and thus able to learn better (and work better) in lighting that approximates daylight as closely as possible."

(KG) "If using fluorescent lights – standard or full-spectrum – be sure to have them electrically shielded with a proper grounding connection."

(RM) "Incandescent light bulbs are a better alternative. LED (light emitting diode) technology looks promising as well."

(MH) "Instead of promoting compact fluorescent light bulbs, governments around the world should be insisting that manufacturers produce light bulbs that are electro-magnetically clean and contain no toxic chemicals. LEDs are a safer option." Unlike compact fluorescent bulbs, LEDs contain no mercury and they work well in cold weather. They may provide a more pleasing light than fluorescents and appear to be the greenest and potentially healthiest option.

(KG) "Watch out for poor quality electronic drivers in LEDs that increase electro-magnetic field emissions and may cause flickers. Models with a proper grounding connection are preferable."

The high cost of LED light production has meant that their use has been limited to commercial and outdoor lighting, but that is changing. Soon they will be more available, and more economical, for use in our homes, offices and schools.

Halogen Lights

The Concern:

(AP) "Low voltage halogen lights are also not recommended as they give off high electric fields, and many have their own built-in transformer. This is usually poorly constructed and gives off very high levels of power-frequency magnetic fields close to them."

Halogen Lights – Safer Solutions:

(KG) "If using low-voltage halogen lights, the transformers should be located away from high-occupancy areas and the wiring shielded. Since most transformers in low-voltage desk lamps emit magnetic fields even when turned off, avoid these. Line-voltage (120V) halogen lamps are better, especially for bedside and desk lamps. See the lighting recommendations in my paper on low-emission office environments: www.buildingbiology.ca/healthyoffice.php"

Night lights

The Concern:

(AP) "There is plenty of strong scientific evidence that shows that even quite low levels of light stop the production of melatonin, a hormonal chemical synthesised in the pineal gland. It, and its associated chemicals, 'mop up' dangerous free-radical damage. There is good evidence that low levels of melatonin increase the likelihood of cancers and other serious health problems developing. It is often your anxiety about seeing your child that starts the 'light at night' habit."

Night Lights – Safer Solutions:

The only type of night light that you should use are the very low power (usually plug mounted) orange or red ones that just glow gently as these colors hardly affect the production of melatonin. White and blue-white lights are likely to stop the pineal gland's production of melatonin for the whole of the night.

(KG) "I am very concerned about light exposure at night, no matter what its color. Darkness is best."

Dimmer Lights

The Concern:

(RM) "Dimmer switches produce elevated magnetic fields and power line transients, which are high frequency noise on the power lines."

Dimmer Lights – Safer Solution:

(RM) "Remove dimmer switches."

(MB) "Get rid of instant-on devices."

(SH) "Do not have dimmer lights or touch-on (clap-on) lamps near where you sit or sleep."

Even if you choose to be wary of cell phones, cordless phones and wireless Internet you are still be exposed to EMR in all kinds of ways that have never occurred to you, and ones that you may not be able to control.

Consider the following.

Medical Technologies

One of Dr. Becker's concerns was that our conventional medical system relies on powerful testing and treatment technologies that may administer high doses of EMR. Dr. William Rea, also a surgeon and a highly respected pioneer in this field, reports that he became electro-sensitive from being immersed many hours a day in the radiation around him.

At what point do the risks begin to outweigh the benefits?

Pre-natal Ultrasound

This snapshot of your unborn child can offer a magical moment for expectant parents, and also crucial medical information. I just want you to know that some experts have advised caution. How it works: ultrasound is a sound wave transmitted in water or biological tissue. A low energy ultrasound is used in medicine as a diagnostic imaging technique, especially in obstetrics.

The Benefits: finding out whether a fetus is growing normally.

The Concern:

Some expectant parents are subjecting their babies to multiple ultrasounds for reasons that aren't medically necessary. The Federal Drug Administration (FDA) in the US, and the Society of Obstetricians and Gynecologists of Canada are among the medical experts who caution:

> Although there have been no fetal abnormalities linked directly to diagnostic ultrasound, it involves targeted energy exposure to the fetus, and there remains a theoretical risk for subtle effects on fetal development.

This is suggested by some biological effects of ultrasound observed at, or near, diagnostic intensities in both human studies and animal models.

Source: Non-medical Use of Ultrasound – SOGC Policy Statement April 2007

There is also concern that some technicians may deliver a stronger exposure than required, or may try to reposition the fetus for a better viewing angle.

(KG) "The sound level of an ultrasound scanner is 100 dB; in the human audible range, this would be comparable to subjecting your fetus to the sound level of a jackhammer at 1 m distance."

Ultrasound Safer Solution:

The experts' recommendation: have ultrasound only when medically necessary.

Dental/Medical X-rays

Electro-magnetic waves at this very high frequency – called ionizing radiation – may damage or kill cells through the production of free radicals.

What are free radicals?

You'll need a small dose of science here if you want to know what this means. The high-energy waves from X-rays interact with DNA in your body tissue and dislodge electrons, splitting the atom into negatively charged electrons and a positively charged ion.

This ion, or free radical, behaves wildly seeking to replace its missing

---

electron. (I once heard this described as 'recently single, seeking a mate'.) The unleashed reaction of free radicals in the body can lead to the disruption of intra-cellular metabolism and interference with DNA repair.

As you may know, many forms of cancer are thought to be the result of free radicals reacting with DNA, resulting in unwanted cell mutations. (Antioxidant nutritional supplements are considered by many physicians to reduce the production of these free radicals.)

Dental X-rays

Again this procedure has its benefits – and risks. I was often told that there was no concern about these levels of radiation. ("Just like a day in the sunshine".) Now I'm not so sure this is true.

Our new family dentist does not have the digital X-ray machine, but I found one office that does, so if any of us need a dental X-ray we go there to have this lower-exposure kind.

How dental X-rays work: a beam of radiation is focused to go through your teeth and onto a small piece of photographic film. Dense structures such as teeth and bones absorb more X-rays than the soft tissues. Cavities and infections will show up as lighter areas because more radiation has passed through them before striking the film.

The Benefit: finding decay and diagnosing periodontal disease in impossible-to-see areas, such as under fillings or between teeth.

The Concern:

While the amount of radiation in any one X-ray is reportedly 'small', exposure is cumulative – it builds up with each one. In the head and neck, areas exposed to dental radiation, X-rays increase the risk of damage to, or cancer of, the lens of the eye, thyroid, salivary glands, bone marrow and skin. Scientists in the UK have found that about 0.6% of the cumulative cancer risk in people under age 75 – about 700 cases per year – could be attributed to diagnostic X-rays. In Japan, which has the highest frequency of diagnostic X-ray exposure in the world, the risk was more than 3%.

Source: The Lancet, Vol. 363, Issue 9406

Dental X-rays – Safer Solutions:

Question your dentist – is the X-ray essential? Why? I switched dentists when one insisted our children needed whole mouth X-rays "on file". Find a practitioner who uses newer digital X-rays, which evidently beam out 90% less radiation.

Medical X-rays – Safer Solutions:

It's a similar situation with medical X-rays, used, among other reasons, to check for broken bones, or in the case of chest X-rays, to diagnose pneumonia. I don't want to scare you away from essential medical tests, but to encourage you to discuss with your practitioner whether there's another way to get the information needed for diagnosis. Again, is this X-ray essential? Do people with recurring sinus infections really need to have their heads X-rayed? What is the effect on their eyes? Brains?

Medical thermography emits nothing – there is no radiation. It only takes an image and these thermal readings can be a useful tool in detecting and monitoring a number of diseases and physical injuries. This FDA approved test can show physiological change and metabolic processes and is used with back injuries, for example. Thermography can also offer early detection of breast abnormalities and monitor changes. This is an option with, or instead of, mammography. More research on the safety and effectiveness of mammograms is needed.

CT and MRI scans

I also hesitate to sound an alarm about these tests, as it seems unlikely anyone would have them unless it was medically crucial – when the benefits would outweigh the risks. Or so I used to think!

Private clinics are now marketing full-body CT and MRI scans to the general public, even those who have no other signs of disease.

Health authorities agree there is no scientific evidence that using these scans on people without symptoms is useful in catching diseases early. If the tests produce suspicious findings, this could lead to having more unnecessary procedures, exploratory surgery, medications, etc.

If the scan shows nothing, you might then ignore signs of an actual illness that can't be detected by scans. And that's before you even consider the potential side effects of the procedures themselves.

The Concern:

In December 2008, American researchers, developing tools to help doctors weigh the risks and benefits of CT (computed tomography) scans, reported that as many as 7 percent of patients from a large U.S. hospital system received enough radiation exposure from scans over the course of their lifetime to slightly increase their risk of cancer.

The researchers raised the concern that repeated scans of people who had cancer could increase the patients' chances of developing another tumor.

And in February 2009 a paper in the Journal of the *American Medical Association* reported that one CT angiogram, widely used by cardiologists to find potentially fatal blockages in heart arteries, could deliver a radiation dose equivalent to 600 chest X-rays.

Researchers caution that whole body CT screening exposes you to radiation levels that up to 1000 times as high as those from an X-ray, increasing your risk of developing radiation-induced cancer.

MRI (magnetic resonance imaging) is a different technology, as you may know. Its powerful magnetic field excites the molecules of the body's tissues, causing the nuclei in these molecules to emit a radio-frequency. The MRI scanner transmits these radio signals to a computer, which translates them into a 3-D image of the area being examined.

Unlike CT scans, or other kinds of X-rays, this process does not involve the highest power – ionizing – radiation. Some companies are marketing MRIs as having 'no radiation'; this is not completely true. And, some people claim they became electro-sensitive only after having had an MRI.

Unnecessary scans could increase the risk of bringing on the very diseases you're worried about and trying to detect early. So the recommendation is to have these tests only when medically necessary. Even if your doctor is ordering them, you have the right to question. And to a second opinion.

Mark Baerlocher, MD, a fellow in interventional radiology at University of California, San Diego, offers his concern about, "the lack of awareness, and the general misinformation regarding the radiation risks associated with Medical Imaging and related exams, and procedures, among both health care professionals and patients." This concern led him to develop the Radiation Passport, a computer program to help patients, physicians, and dentists track lifetime exposures and better understand the risks. One can look up the estimated effective radiation dose associated with a given Medical Imaging exam or procedure, and the associated estimated risk of developing cancer due to that radiation.

Medical Scans – Safer Solutions:

Cardiologists say CT angiograms are indispensable in some cases. I was relieved to read that techniques are being developed to reduce the amount of radiation given in these valuable tests. Some physicians who practice complementary medicine recommend a protocol to reduce the impact of X-rays and scans. See *Prescription for Nutritional Healing,* Avery, New York, by James Balch, MD and Phyllis A. Balch, CNC.

Other Exposures:

Radio-frequency ID tags/wristbands

Wireless chips are already everywhere: in tags on clothing in stores, in security access cards, some passports, tollbooths, library books and bus passes. Recently, I saw little units being handed out at a pharmacy prescription counter so the staff could beep people when their prescriptions were ready. I walked past the beeper station quite quickly.

Many of these devices only emit signals when they're run through a scanner. But the ones that are causing more concern are those that send out signals constantly.

How they work:

The chips "communicate" with each other by generating radio frequencies. In hospitals they're used to track medical supplies, equipment, and even people. One hospital in Israel was using RFID wristbands on babies in the neonatal ICU, to make sure each preemie was fed from a container of his or her own mother's milk.

The Benefit:

Better inventory control, faster service. In hospitals, RFID bracelets can help keep track of people with dementia, for instance.

The Concern: According to a study published in the June 2008 Journal of the American Medical Association, tests show these devices may interfere with pacemakers, ventilators, IV pumps and anesthesia machines. And even though evidence exists that tumors can develop at the site of implantation, some pets are still tagged this way. Why?

ID Tags – Safer Solutions:

Hospitals should check all new technology, especially wireless chips, to make sure they don't interfere with medical equipment, and should know about potential adverse biological effects – including cardiac ones. Be aware of this if you have an implanted defibrillator or pacemaker.

Airport Security Scanners – Your Dignity or Your DNA?

How they work:

Metal detectors can't locate plastic explosives so now there are more invasive methods: millimeter wave scanners that use non-ionizing radiation and the more intense backscatter X-ray technology that uses ionizing levels. These scans produce digital images of our body, and any weapons or explosives. There are privacy and health concerns.

The Benefit:

Avoiding the dreaded "enhanced" pat down, speeding up security screening, and theoretically keeping us safer. Everyone wants safe skies. However, this technology may not have been properly screened!

The Concern:

We are told that "the scanners are safe," the low level emissions are "within safety standards" and lower than what we receive from "cosmic radiation during a flight, or being in the earth's magnetic fields." However, natural-source radiation is more diffuse, usually goes right through us, and we've adapted to it. Artificial radiation from scanners is more focused – like a laser beam. We already know about the safety standards. And Professor Olle Johansson questions,

"If airport scanners are safe, then there must be peer review-based scientific publications clearly showing it. If not, then you must ask why not?" Dr. Sinatra queries, "Are there any adverse effects in patients with vulnerable hearts, or in patients with pacemakers and defibrillators?" Our advisory board, Doctors for Safer Skies, is asking these questions, and requesting accurate answers and to see the evidence of safety.

The biochemist Dr. David Agard and others from the University of California urge caution, and Alasdair Philips tells us, "The key point is the bombarding of the skin with a mass of high-energy electrons. That may, or may not be a significant problem, but there has been almost no work done to test it on animals (or humans) at these relatively low energy levels. This technology should not be used until it has been shown over several years not to cause cancer-related problems."

Skin cancer is one concern as the dose is concentrated in the skin and underlying tissue. And eyes, testicles and breast tissue are vulnerable. Dr. Henry Lai has found DNA damage from non-ionizing radiation and Dr. N.P. Singh, and others, from ionizing levels. There's also concern about effects on pregnant women and damage to reproductive DNA.

There's increased risk for flight crews who have high occupational exposure and frequent flyers – both groups pass often through security. And there's wireless radiation at airports, and in-flight Wi-Fi on planes.

Security Scanners – Safer Solutions:

You may have to put up with the indignity of the intrusive pat down to avoid being scanned. If you are electro-sensitive or pregnant, have a pacemaker or heart condition, or have had skin cancer, inform security staff that you need this alternative; also a prudent choice with children.

(KG) "It's not just scanners; flying increases radiation exposure. During pregnancy or with babies, it is best not to travel by airplane, certainly not on an intercontinental flight. The ionizing radiation exposure from the cosmic radiation is rather high, especially at higher altitudes."

Smart Meter ™

A Smart Meter is a remote way the electric, gas or water company reads a meter. There are several ways these meters work. Some use radio waves that can cause some people to feel ill. Contrary to what your utility company may tell you, technical experts report these emit very high levels of RF – certainly strong enough to cause health problems. Find out what method is used for yours. If it is a radio wave method, ask that the SmartMeter be replaced with a regular mechanical meter. You may have to pay a bit more, but your exposure is less, and given the evidence of adverse health effects, and some people's medical electro-sensitivity, we should have a choice – a right to health issue to fight for.

Wired Devices

Now let's look at the devices from the lower frequencies – the first part of the Spectrum. (As you may remember, we examined the third category – X-rays, etc. – in our last section with the Risk Survey information.)

Computers

Computer screens are an EMR issue.

As you may know, the older standard monitors, with cathode ray tubes (CRT), emit high levels all around them. These are the curved back chunky kinds, sadly often found in school computer labs.

All CRT monitors give off higher fields at the back and sides. Always sit more than a metre (39 inches) from the rear. I have been told by EMR technicians that if you have a bank of computers, it is better to put them back to back to minimize this exposure.

Magnetic fields travel through walls, so watch the use of the next room (for instance, don't let it be your child's sleeping room).

Smaller monitors are not necessarily better than large ones, because the field's strength depends more on the internal design than on the screen size.

The flat LCD screen is a better choice. I chose the low-tech LCD model that had small speakers and no other frills. It also has a good-sized screen so that I could place it far back from where I sit - more than an arm's length away.

(SH) "Infrared computer gear is okay, including some keyboard and mouse connections."

With the keyboard, again you want the wired, not wireless. The same applies to the mouse. Also, I have heard that the optical mouse, because of its design, has a higher electro-magnetic field than the laser variety. I am using a corded laser mouse.

If I find ones with proven lower EMR levels, I will post this information on our website.

Laptop computers

The Concern:

(AP) "These handy computers can emit significant levels of electric fields from the back illumination and scanning processes. When run from the plug-in adapters, they can give off very high electric fields next to the keyboard and display, of several hundred volts/metre."

Not too long ago, a woman contacted me when she heard about this book, asking if the numbness in her legs might be caused by sitting for long periods with her wireless laptop on her lap. Evidently she did a trial of sitting in the same position for the same amount of time without the laptop, with no numbness in her legs.

When I gave her the short story about effects of wireless technology, she responded abruptly, "Oh, I couldn't do without that. I'm a writer."

Laptops – Safer Solutions:

(KG) "Laptops also give off very high magnetic fields at close range where you have your hands at the keypad, therefore it is better to use a laptop with an external keyboard whenever possible."

(AP) "Charge laptop computers away from where you sit, and then run them off their internal recharged batteries, or with a grounded power supply."

Remember what I said about proximity?

This might sound contradictory, but all of the experts say don't use a laptop on your lap. Whenever possible, place it on a desk or table or with some other surface between the computer and your body.

I have also learned that electrical devices react with each other, even through walls, so you don't want to sit between your computer and in the direct line of fire with another strong electrical device, like a television, for example.

There are many good reasons to limit computer time; as you know gazing absentmindedly, or even mindfully, at a computer screen can be a factor in a myriad of eye symptoms and conditions. Again, there is a real concern with the amount of time children spend staring into computer/video screens.

Encourage your children to get outside, whenever you can. Maybe even

wander outside with them. Doesn't matter if it's not a bright sunny day.

As Richard Louv wisely remarks in *Last Child in the Woods,* "There's no bad weather, just wearing the wrong clothes."

With so much time sitting at a computer, many of us suffer from repetitive strain injuries, such as carpal tunnel syndrome, headaches and muscle pains in the low back, shoulders and neck. All in all, it's not the best activity for our wellbeing.

On my computer I keep a sticky note reminding me to:

Stretch.   Breathe.   Blink.   Take a Break.   Get outside.

In your office at home or at work, there are many electrical devices you may want to move farther away from you, downgrade to a lower tech version, or remove altogether.

Other office equipment

How many times a day do you see people clustered around a huge, humming photocopier waiting for a long document?

The concern:

(AP) "Photocopiers give off quite high levels of EMFs from the motor. It would be advisable not to stand immediately next to the motor while it is working. Photocopiers also emit significant levels of ozone, and should always be in a well-ventilated room, or in a corridor. Volatile organic compounds (VOCs) are released, which increase with warmth, and double-sided copying. VOCs are given off even when the photocopier is not working, but is still switched on."

(AP) "Printers, scanners and fax machines can all give off significant levels of EMF near them, and some laser printers also release ozone.

Office Equipment – Safer Solutions:

It's obviously best to place printers, fax machines, copiers etc. as far away as possible from where you sit, and don't stand next to them while they're in operation. This is the basic recommendation with all electrical equipment.

If you have a wireless printer, consider replacing it with a wired one. Ink-jet printers are more ecologically friendly than laser printers and do not give off ozone.

Entertainment Devices

The Concern and Safer Solutions:

(AP) "**Televisions** give off high magnetic and electric fields up to 1.5 metres away (about 4 feet). Remember that magnetic fields travel through walls. EMR from **digital TVs** is not much different in level from older analog models, though some people with EHS say that they are more affected by them. Children should not sit close to any size television. Watch TV, including plasma screens, from a minimum of 2 metres (7 feet) away.

Plasma screens give off high levels of electric fields. Use the main switch on the set to switch off the television. Some types of remote control leave the TV on standby and it continues to consume up to a quarter of the energy it uses when switched on."

(KG) "LCD TV screens usually have much lower EMF emissions than plasma TV screens."

These days, all TV and video remote controls work using very low-power infrared light, and pose no problems.

(RM) "Some high tech remote controls do use RF but are only transmitting when buttons are pushed."

Analog TV reception signals are relatively low power and are believed to have few biological effects.

(KG) "It is true that digital TV radiation seems to be more biologically active than analog TV. But if you happen to live in the vicinity of an analog TV tower, levels are so high that this will also cause major adverse health impacts."

(RM) "TV reception signals are switching to digital and these will pose a health threat."

Digital TV receivers can give off high electric fields if the TV system, or satellite decoder, is not connected to the building's electrical grounding wire. Most TVs, video recorders and satellite systems are not grounded when you buy them, as they only have a two-wire power cord, rather than a grounded three-prong plug. Walls will give some protection from the electric fields; windows are less effective at screening them.

DVD and video players and recorders have transformers, in their power supplies, which can generate strong magnetic fields.

TV, video and Hi-Fi microwave transmitter boxes, used to transmit pictures and sound from your main entertainment system to all other rooms in the house with a suitable receiver box, should be avoided. They are another source of microwave exposure in your home environment.

Personal portable music players

(RM) "Personal music players can affect the electrically sensitive even if not Wi-Fi. Recommendations are to keep electronics off of the body."

Note: The new 'improved' wireless-enabled music players are not recommended for the obvious reason that the listener is now exposed to wireless radiation. Listening to music from a laptop, which is wirelessly connected, is also not recommended.

Electric Heating Pads, Electric Blankets, Electric Mattress Pads, etc.

Electric blankets and heating pads seem comforting, and health-enhancing. Or at least, we think they are. Remember my surrounding my dear mother with this electric warmth to keep her sluggish circulation moving?

The Concern:

(RM) "These heating devices have wires threaded through them, and electricity is used to create heat. I think it is easy to see the issues when they are plugged in and turned on. While operational, extreme levels of AC Electric and possibly AC Magnetic Fields can exist.

If they are turned off and still plugged in there still may be a high electric field because of the mere presence of electricity on its power cord. And the wires that run throughout the items can act as an antenna for radio waves and also re-radiate other electric fields from other sources."

Dr. Andrew Weil, (AW), a respected physician and health educator advises on his website: www.drweil.com:

(AW) "Household appliances such as heating pads, electric blankets and mattress covers, plug-in hair dryers, computers, and coffee-makers all generate EMFs that surround electrical equipment, power cords, and power lines.

Some research has suggested that exposure to low-level magnetic fields emitted by such appliances as hair dryers, electric blankets and electric razors can damage DNA in brain cells.

The data come from a study in rats at the University of Washington (conducted by Henry Lai, PhD) which found DNA damage in animals exposed to a 60 hertz field for 24 hours; more damage was found after 48 hours."

Electric Blankets, etc. – Safer Solutions:

On his website, Dr. Weil also suggests: "Because we can't say for sure that electro-magnetic fields pose no risks, I would advise you to use a non-electric heating pad, such as one that you warm up in hot water."

(RM) "Find non-electrical methods for heating your bed, like an organic wool/cotton comforter. And it is recommended to keep wires and metal away from the sleeping area. Also use a non-metallic mattress and foundation like natural latex with an organic cotton/wool topper."

Your Sleep Zone – Another Reminder

As we have mentioned, all experts advise making our sleeping areas electronic-free zones, as much as we can. This is especially important if anyone is vulnerable due to age, illness, electro-sensitivity etc., or who is experiencing any of the symptoms or conditions we have listed as being related to EMR exposure.

If anyone is having trouble sleeping, lowering the levels, as much as possible, is strongly recommended. Most electro-sensitive people have sleep disorders. Meters can help determine the best place in the house to sleep and to monitor the effectiveness of interventions.

While having a low EMR sleep zone is very important for us all, it is *crucial* for babies and young children.

Baby's Room – Must be a low-EMR environment

(AP) "Arrange your baby's sleeping area so that he or she is at least a metre (3.25 feet) from the nearest electric appliance and about that far away from the wall. Don't use a dimmer switch to provide a light in the baby's sleeping room, unless it is well away from the baby's head. Ensure the bulb it is lighting is red or orange, not white or bluish."

You know, of course, that it's prudent to avoid electronics in a baby's, or young child's room. These precautions include avoiding plugged-in clocks [use battery ones], fluorescent lights [use incandescents] and cordless phones [use corded ones.] And it's best to avoid digital baby monitors – see the next few pages for details. It is especially important if you are pregnant, or want to be, or if you have a newborn or young children in the house, to also make sure your Internet access is wired, not wireless, as a wireless router radiates for hundreds of feet (metres). Cautions also include avoiding exposure to cell phone radiation and microwave ovens, as you know by now. Your whole family will benefit.

(RM) "Be aware of what is in the room below or beside the baby's sleeping area. I find many houses have fluorescent light fixtures mounted underneath the bedrooms, which may be on when the children are sleeping. Make sure no one, especially a child, is sleeping close to appliances in adjoining rooms. Smart Meters are also a concern."

(CA) "I recommend not having a fuse box, television, fridge or other electronics on the other side of the wall from a crib or child's bed."

Baby Monitors

The Concern:

Now that you know a lot about the health hazards of wireless radiation and digital DECT cordless phones, imagine this kind of radiation-emitting device near a newborn. If you know parents who have a digital/wireless monitor in their child's room, please let them know. Let's alert the companies that make these, and the retail and online stores that sell them. When they hear that we won't buy digital/wireless monitors they will bring back the safer analog/wired ones.

Larry Gust comments: "The baby monitor signal used to be run through the house electrical wiring to where mom or dad were listening. Then 'progress' was made and the monitor went wireless using analog radio waves. This was okay as long as the monitor was not placed within six feet of baby. Then came more 'progress' using digital radio signals. A component of this signal is unhealthy for the cells in the baby's body, and yours. Now virtually all baby monitors are wireless and digital – emitting digital microwave radiation throughout the baby's room."

(KG) "Digital baby monitors measured one foot away (30cm) emit RF levels up to 20,000 (microwatts per sq. metre) – very high levels."

A Factor in SIDS?

I read a report about an increase in sudden infant death syndrome – tragic deaths. Pre-natal EMR exposure has been shown to cause harm to organs of the developing fetus. Could this and/or exposure to the infant from digital baby monitors, mobile phones and Wi-Fi in the home be a factor in SIDS? Is anyone looking into this, or monitoring the cumulative effects on a fetus, or infant, of unprecedented EMR levels? Until the research is done, we need to take protective action.

A grandmother who read this book, with increasing horror, evidently, told me that she insisted steps be taken to reduce EMR in her grandchildren's environment. The children's parents balked at the perceived loss of convenience but soon adapted, and she reports all are well and sleeping better. Never underestimate a determined granny.

Baby Monitors – Safer Solutions:

(AP) "Avoid the 2.4 GHz (gigaHertz) and 5.8 GHz digital baby monitors. Use the old fashioned plug-in or analog type. As long as the analog monitor unit is six feet away from the baby, it does not appear to present a risk. Find older ones at garage sales, thrift stores, eBay, etc. Look for the antenna to be about 6 inches or more long. If the antenna is not visible, or is one inch or less, the unit is the 2.4 GHz or 5.8 GHz and should be avoided."

Baby Sensor Pads/Crib Bedding

(AP) "Sensor pads are put under the mattress to monitor the baby's breathing. One well-known UK make was found to produce significant levels of pulsing microwaves around the baby's body."

(LG) "Some parents use sensor pads as extra protection against crib death. Wireless systems are a problem and the type of the baby's bedding is also an important concern. Dr Jim Sprott, a New Zealand scientist, states that SIDS is caused by toxic gases. These gases can be generated from the mattress when a fungus, that commonly grows in bedding, interacts with fire retardant chemicals that are added to mattresses (Richardson 1994).

Depending on conditions, these heavier-than-air gases, generated by the fungus acting on the retardants, are concentrated in a thin layer on the baby's mattress, or dissipated into the surrounding atmosphere. If a baby breathes or absorbs a lethal dose of the gases, the central nervous system shuts down, stopping breathing and heart function. These gases can fatally poison a baby, without waking the sleeping baby and without any struggle. A normal autopsy would not reveal any sign that the baby was poisoned (Sprott 1996 & 2000)."

(LG) "Eliminate all sources of phosphorus, arsenic and antimony from mattresses. Putting the mattresses in a gas-impermeable cover made from high-grade polyethylene can prevent exposure to these gases plus insuring that bedding used on top of a covered mattress does not contain any phosphorus, arsenic or antimony.

Dr. Sprott specifies a pure cotton flannelette under blanket, with only cotton, or poly-cotton sheets and woolen, or cotton blankets over the baby. No other bedding should be used. Do not use synthetic sheets or blankets, duvet, sleeping bag, or sheepskin.

Baby Sensor Pads/Bedding – Safer Solutions:

The simple, and safe, choice is a wired system. When I visited a family with a child at risk, we tested their wireless sensor pad and the RF readings were high. On our recommendation, they had just purchased a wired one; the RF readings were zero. An easy choice once you know.

Crib toys

Battery-operated stuffies/toys look so cuddly – some even emit a range of soothing sounds – but are they safe?

(LG) "The level of radiation is very small. Yet, newborns are in a critical phase of life. I would not give these to an infant."

(AP) "I would have these toys outside, not inside, of the bed/cot. And I see no good reason that sound generators need to be built inside a young child's toy. Be aware that increasing numbers of these toys have a microprocessor inside that will generate some EMF very close by."

Hair Dryers, Electric Razors

The Concern:

If you are a barber or professional hair stylist, this is a significant concern. Remember the factors of intensity, proximity and duration?

Dr. Henry Lai cautioned:

> Data suggest that the effects of EMF exposure are cumulative and may build up in humans over time as a result of repeated brief use of common plug-in appliances. I suggest limiting exposure to as little time as possible, particularly with devices used close to the body.

(AP) "The motor of a hair dryer gives off very high fields near the handle, dropping only a little at normal drying distances (6 to 18 inches). The fields are slightly higher on high heat, than low heat. Any metal hairpins will increase exposure. It's recommended not to use hair dryers etc. after 7 pm. High magnetic fields near the head in the evening could interfere with the production of melatonin – needed for sleep – by the pineal gland for the rest of that night.

The heating units for electric hair curlers give off significant levels. Sit away from the heating unit while it is still working. When you have removed the curlers, switch off the heating unit.

Hair curling tongs and flattening irons give off quite high fields. It is best to use them with care.

Sitting under a hooded hair dryer regularly is not recommended as they emit a high field. Metal pins will increase EMR exposure.

Electric razors also give off high fields. Again, this is more of a concern with professionals who are handling them all day."

Having read this far, no doubt you are now leaping ahead to your own safer solutions considering proximity, duration etc. There are also lower-EMF hair dryers advertised. What meter would you use to test the field around them? Yes, the Gauss meter that measures the non-communicating type of radiation.

Hair dryers, Electric Razors – Safer Solutions:

(AW) "The strength of EMF falls off exponentially as distance from the source increases. So hold the hair dryer farther away."

Non-electric razors are an option if you are concerned about this exposure.

Electric Alarm Clocks/Clock radios

Imagine my consternation when I saw a fully-loaded bedside unit: a sleek silver wireless router, alarm clock and CD combo unit for sale, in a pharmacy, no less!

The Concern:

If a plugged in clock, or any other electronic gadget, is lying within a few feet of your head all night, you're receiving that exposure when your body most needs a low-EMR environment. This is not a minor concern and may have significant impact on our health over time.

Clocks – Safer Solutions:

(SH) "Plugged-in clocks, radios etc. should be kept at least 6 feet away from where you sleep."

The best option is a battery-operated alarm clock. The next best is a small electric alarm clock placed at least six feet from you; those of us older than 40 may have to get one with larger numbers!

Other Electric Equipment

Hot Tubs/Whirlpool Baths – Yes, these tubs of hot swirling water are relaxing, but we should know the powerful motors produce electro-magnetic fields.

(AP) "Most have pumps and motors built in to the base resulting in high EMR exposure as you take a bath. It's recommended that the pumps and motors are at least half a metre (roughly 2 feet) away from the bath.

Sunbeds emit high electric and magnetic fields, as well as possibly dangerous levels of ultraviolet radiation. And many can give off five times as much UVA as would be expected from bright sunlight at the equator.

These will increase your risk of developing skin cancer, especially if you are fair-skinned.

Sunlamps – the EMR is not as high as sunbeds, but like sunbeds they give off ultraviolet light – a form of radiation that we know causes skin cancers.

Exercise machines – Motors (such as those used to power treadmills) give off high magnetic fields. You are usually not that close to the motor so they are generally not a problem. The exercise is probably more beneficial than the small level of potential risk.

Vibrating muscle toners emit both electric and magnetic fields. Probably all right if you are not electrically sensitive or pregnant."

(KG) "Depending an the device, muscle-toning machines can emit substantial amounts of EMF. A rebounder is definitely a safer option."

(AP) "**TENS** (transcutaneous electrical nerve stimulation) machines are used for chronic pain control and muscle stimulation. They work by passing short pulses of electrical energy though parts of the body. Not recommended if you are electrically sensitive."

Power Tools

The problem here is much the same as with devices like hair dryers and electric razors. If you're a professional, using high-power versions all day, it's more of concern than if you're just doing the occasional odd job around the house. It may be possible to find some models with shielded power cords.

Obviously, if you're pregnant, electro-sensitive, recovering from cancer or otherwise immune-compromised, you may want to consider your use of these.

Electrical – Wiring and Fuse Boxes

The Concern:

This was a surprise to me. Even when plugged-in things are not turned on, they emit an electrical field. This includes the miles of wiring in buildings.

You can test these lower frequency exposures, from the first window of our Spectrum, with a reliable electric field meter. It is worth it to have a professional testing of your home, office and school for these fields as the radiation can 'pool' in spots and the professionals know where, and how, to test for these fields. And their instruments are highly sensitive and reliable.

An EMR-qualified electrician can advise you and do the work on your house wiring – for instance installing demand switches to turn off circuits when they're not being used. Then you can retest on your own to assess the effectiveness of your interventions. This is certainly something to keep in mind when you're building a new house or about to do a major renovation.

(KG) "Demand switches should only be installed if proper testing was done first to identify the contributing circuits. To my knowledge, there is no consumer electric-field probe that would give you reliable readings.

Body voltage testing can give you false readings, depending on the electrical conductivity of surrounding building materials e.g. in close range to grounding pads, stucco on wire mesh, metal roofs, etc."

Electrical Wiring – Safer Solutions

Building or renovating?

(CA) "Ideally, it is preferable and far less expensive and problematic to have an EMR professional create a low EMR wiring design and implementation – before the construction stage – using shielded cable throughout the building. This eliminates all electric fields from wiring sources."

Fuse Boxes – Safer Solutions:

(RM) "Locate household power meters and fuse boxes away from main living areas. They may be a source of high magnetic fields."

Power Cords

(RM) "Do not have power cords near your feet, or under your bed. Where power cords are necessary, use shielded ones as they reduce the EMF levels drastically."

Power Lines

If you live close to power lines, you should test inside, and outside, your house and property to know how much radiation you're being exposed to. Best to hire a professional, or get a Gauss meter and do it yourself.

Experts warn that these high-voltage power lines should not be close to schools, hospitals, or where people live.

Environmental health consultant Stan Hartman tells us:

> People should also know that neighborhood power lines are a concern, as they can have stronger fields than huge towering transmission lines. Be sure to check the lines at different times of day and on different days.

Here is an example of what we are up against. In British Columbia, the official response to Moms Against Power Lines, from a chief medical health officer, was "I've been following this thing for my 35 years in public health and there is no real danger."

Power Lines – Safer Solutions:

Ideally, you choose a neighborhood after you've checked out the radiation levels emitted from cell phone base stations, or radio or ham broadcast antennas, radar, or some power lines. Stan Hartman suggests the only solution is to paint all the walls and doors with shielding paint, and cover the windows with metal screening or metallic sunshield or shielding fabric. There's more about these products and associated cautions later in this section.

(KG) "If properly installed, metal screenings/shielding fabric could protect from the electric field exposure (and potentially from wireless transmitters if specified for it). One of the major components of power line emissions is magnetic fields, which the shielding paints and metal screenings would not address. The safest solution for power lines is to keep sufficient distance."

Vehicles

Electric/Hybrid Cars

Unfortunately, the energy-saving strategy of hybrid cars may have significant risks for human health. A hybrid vehicle combines a regular internal combustion engine and an electric motor powered by batteries. When you start the car, and at low speeds, the car runs just with the electric motor and battery. At high speeds the gasoline engine kicks in. The electric motor and batteries help the conventional engine work more efficiently, so far less fuel is used compared to even very efficient gas-powered vehicles. A good goal.

Electric/Hybrid Cars – The Concern:

However, these vehicles have big battery packs just behind the rear seat, with cables running underneath the passengers toward the front of the car. Some drivers have used Gauss meters to check inside their hybrid vehicles for the EMR levels from the flow of electrical current to the motor. They reported very high levels – hundreds of times higher than our scientists consider safe.

There are also anecdotal reports of drivers of hybrids complaining of new health problems including rising blood pressure, excessive fatigue while driving, and other symptoms of electro-hypersensitivity. I hear they are developing hybrid trucks and buses – very big batteries. Good for global warming, but what about the health of the occupants?

(LG) "The magnetic fields are approximately 10 times higher in hybrids than in conventional vehicles, depending on the measurement location in the car."

The back seat reading can be extremely high. Is this really where you want to put your baby's car seat?

Hybrid Cars – Safer Solutions:

Shielding for the batteries. Unlike in mobile communications, there are no information-carrying radio waves here, so the batteries can be completely covered with a special metal that blocks the EMR, without disrupting the efficiency of the battery.

(KG) "In order to block the magnetic fields from the batteries, the current-carrying wires would also have to be shielded."

EMR in your gasoline-powered car?

Even in the non-hybrid vehicles, there are hundreds of electrical devices producing strong fields. Our car has electrically-heated seats. I used to think this was a great winter feature.

The Concern:

(KG) "Most cars emit substantial amounts of magnetic fields. Depending on the tires and the location of electronics and wiring, exposure levels can vary greatly in conventional cars, and can be just as bad as in hybrid cars."

(AP) "Cars have electrical and electronic equipment (power wiring, fan motors, computerised controls and dashboards) that can disturb electrically sensitive people. The front seat can be a particular risky area.

Some upmarket cars have electronic control units under (or even as a part of) the driver's seat. These will give off high magnetic fields. Also worth checking is whether the angle and position of car seats are electrically controlled. These have higher EMF/EMR than mechanically operated seats."

(LG) "Other features in conventional cars can cause discomfort e.g. an air conditioning system control that sits in the ceiling right above the driver's head and puts out a high magnetic field. This has given some a blinding headache. When the cause was discovered and the equipment disconnected, the headache never returned."

(CA) "In gas-fuelled vehicles, spark plugs firing repeatedly a few feet from occupants causes RF exposure. Many EMR-sensitive people react to this. Diesel cars without spark plugs do not have this problem."

Newer conventional vehicles also present more exposure than the older cars do, because of the on-board computers, and other high-tech additions.

Non-hybrid Cars – Safer Solutions:

If you're considering buying a new vehicle, or when you're booking a rental, it's preferable to get one with as few electronic bells and whistles as possible. Choose your car carefully, preferably using a meter (see Resources at the end of the book) to detect the fields. And, to be mindful of our environment, you can always opt for the most fuel-efficient conventional vehicles, limit your amount of driving, limit speeding, carpool etc.

Global Positioning Systems (GPS)

Have you been reading this and wondering if there's going to be any GOOD news? Well, here's some. I have recently learned that the on-board GPS is *not* so much of a concern, until it gets 'amped-up' for other sending and receiving functions?

(LG) "The GPS is a receiving-only device emitting a small amount of radiation – more like a radio."

However we are being exposed to more and more wireless radiation as we travel.

Wireless on the road and by rail?

Someone contacted me recently to ask about wireless access in vehicles (via Bluetooth-like systems). Evidently, some new cars have this built right into the sound systems, but are activated with the ignition so you do not have the option to drive the car without being exposed to this kind of radiation. A confined metal space, experts advise us, can increase the harmful effects of EMR.

One of my neighbors was horrified when I told her about this:

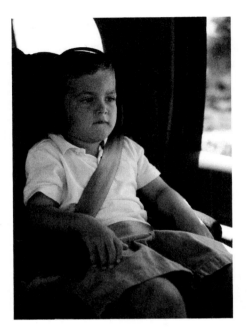

You're not serious? There was just a huge study showing wireless is safe. Our new high-tech car is outfitted with wireless access. The kids think this is very cool.

We even got them wireless headphones.

I thought we were doing the right thing, and that the onboard Wi-Fi and DVD player were going to be so handy. This is frustrating. How are we supposed to know?

If you have traveled lately by train, or a long-distance bus, you know that many are now "wireless hot spots" whether you want it or not. The health effects are just one of the concerns; as you will see in the next section, this kind of radiation has been shown to affect cognitive abilities including reaction time.

Having the conductor, or driver, texting is an obvious distraction, but making transportation vehicles wireless presents other hazards. This is particularly worrying in a high-speed train, or in an aircraft.

Airplane Travel - Wireless in the Sky?

Alasdair Philips, the electrical engineer heading Powerwatch, has done onboard testing of the electro-magnetic fields in aircraft cabins.

He warns:

> Some airlines are planning in-flight mobile phone and Wi-Fi service. They are installing a picocell base station – effectively, a small mobile phone mast – onboard the aircraft.

> Passengers web-browsing and video streaming greatly increase the RF levels in the cabin.

Many experts are seriously alarmed by this. A group of European physicians, the German Environmental Physician Initiative, headed by Dr. Scheiner, wrote a letter (the complete letter is in Resources) to many airline companies about how in-flight wireless can affect the passengers, and the crew – including the crew's cognitive functions. Now that's a scary thought.

Yes, the proponents of this technology have tested the effect on the aircraft navigation systems. No problem, evidently. Have they, however, tested the impact on the pilot and other air crew?

Radiation from Mobile Phones and Reaction Time

Dr. Hans Scheiner:

> I have talked with a pilot who explained that the technical problems – potential interference with onboard navigational equipment – have been solved. However, there's a biological problem to consider. There are not yet any scientific studies of the biological effects on the crew and passengers, but there is enough evidence to cause concern.
>
> While the airplane is moving at an altitude between 8,000 and 12,000 metres, a reduced air pressure occurs inside of the plane, which equals the air pressure of 2,000 – 3,000 metres outside. Therefore the breakage of the blood-brain barrier is more likely because of the lack of oxygen and the well known altitude sickness.
>
> The severe consequences of the brain and nerve damages and safety of passengers are very concerning especially those of the pilots, because they are already highly exposed from radar. The symptoms caused by high frequencies like headaches, drowsiness, vertigo, nausea are often connected with loss of hearing and vision; lack of concentration and memorization are in this context known as the "Microwave-Syndrome" (Johnson-Liakouris, 1998, Mild 1998, Santini 2001, 2002, 2003, Navarro, Oberfeld 2003).

A British lab found that reaction time is much longer when someone is exposed to the high frequencies from Wi-Fi and mobile phones.

This is particularly a concern with the pilot's reaction time, when these high frequencies open the blood-brain barrier. This could become a cause of an aviation accident.

Some Canadian researchers at the University of Toronto also found that drivers of vehicles were nearly five times more likely to have an accident when people were using mobile phones in the car.

Remember the list of EMR exposure symptoms: difficulty focusing, concentrating, and staying on task. Cardiac irregularities, unexplained anxiety, and other symptoms are never good at 37 thousand feet. More air rage incidents?

And remember the experts cautioning us that radiation is greatly magnified in a confined metal space, one that is already high exposure.

Alasdair Philips reveals:

> Planes are not an EMF friendly environment even now. Most have in-flight video screens built into the back of each seat. These are a source of high-frequency fields both for the people watching the screen and for those whose seat it is fitted into.

> The personal lights above the seats in a plane are often high-frequency fluorescent lights and can be sources of significant electric fields. Turn yours off.

With added wireless Internet, the RF radiation will bounce up and down the cabin 'metal tube'. There are also signals from various plane transponders mounted under the fuselage which make their way up into the cabin at surprisingly high levels.

Many planes also have an emergency Iridium phone system that is internally active all the time they are in the air, with active handsets at both ends of the plane using a pulsing DECT (digital) cordless phone like signal 24-7.

There was a tragic story of a co-pilot who had a mental breakdown over the mid-Atlantic, and was carried off the plane yelling, "You can just email me". This unfortunate incident could have nothing to do with radiation exposure.

Yes, people are probably clamoring to use their personal electronics onboard. Airline marketing departments take note: Don't you think that most people value being safe in the sky more than convenience?

Airline litigation departments: think of the ramifications if there's an incident attributed to this, and it is proven that no one pre-tested the acute, or long-term, effects of this radiation on the cognitive functions of pilots. And airline companies ignored medical warnings.

I used to work in the aviation industry doing programs for air traffic controllers and pilots, and I know what kind of stress they are under without this added load. I was also a member of the Canadian Aviation Tribunal. I predict we will see a reversal in this policy when airlines realize the risks, and when passengers and the well organized pilots' unions are better informed.

We need preventive action, not an incident.

WASHINGTON, October 2009 (Reuters) — "Pilots of a jetliner that overshot its destination by 150 miles last week told U.S. investigators they became distracted during an extended discussion of crew scheduling that included their use of personal laptops."

Evidently, their airline 'offers wireless Internet on most flights'. Having read what our experts have suggested about how this radiation can affect cognitive abilities, and remembering how microwaves ricochet in an enclosed metal space, are you also wondering what effect the wireless system might have on a flight crew's gap of attention?

If you know any pilots, flight attendants, air traffic controllers, or airline

company executives, please alert them to this potentially disastrous wireless wake-up call.

I am trying my best to get the word out but the company's answer is usually, "The passengers are demanding this onboard convenience."

Remember the children holding the sign, "Is it worth the risk?"

I have worked with many pilot groups and have great respect for their professionalism. No one cares more about flight safety than they do. We should listen more to their concerns.

Here's a quote by "Ask The Pilot" from salon.com:

> Cockpit hardware and software use radio transmissions for a number of tasks. Whether transmitting, receiving or simply sitting idle, cell phones are able to garble these signals. As you might expect, aircraft electronics are

---

designed and shielded with this interference in mind. This should mitigate any ill effects, and to date there are no proven cases where a cell phone has adversely affected the outcome of a flight. But you never know, and in some situations – for instance, in the presence of old or faulty shielding – it's possible that a telephone could bring about some sort of anomaly.

Anomaly?

Security is also an issue, advises a computer consultant, as the passengers could well include hackers with nothing to do except poke around your files. There are also concerns that online connectivity in the skies could facilitate communication between terrorists planning, or co-ordinating, an attack.

And there are privacy issues. Who wants loud, endless chatter, or worse, on nearby mobile devices.

If you are electro-sensitive it may be difficult already for you to travel. As more of us become electro-sensitive, we will need special areas set aside in airports that are "Wireless Free".

Safer Solutions? Let's lobby the airlines, and regulatory agencies, to test the biological effects of accumulative EMR exposure on flight crews, and passengers, not just the technical equipment.

Another Aviation and Wireless Issue?

In 2003 the SARS virus, and in 2009 the swine flu epidemic, sped around the world, often by air travel, threatening a global pandemic. As wireless radiation has been shown to impair the immune system, we must consider the impact of millions of people traveling in wireless-enabled planes, and trains – confined metal spaces – during these outbreaks.

Hotel/Motel Accommodations

Medical spas, yoga centers and roadside motels are advertising "free wireless Internet". As more of us request *wireless-free* accommodations, this will change. Look for places that at least restrict the wireless to public spaces, and provide only hard-wired access in the sleeping rooms. You will sleep better, think more clearly, and be more relaxed, the experts advise us, if your room is not in a wireless zone. It's also wise to unplug cordless phones, or at least move them away from the sleeping area. Most places have corded phones for use during power outages.

Talk to the places you visit and ask if they provide wireless-free accommodations. And for all of our safety, ask for a Wi-Fi-free flight. As you know, the marketplace responds to us, the consumers.

Safer-Technology?

Shielding electrical wiring, better lighting etc. are a few ways to reduce our EMR exposure. Many of our contributing experts are also calling out for the development of safer – less harmful – devices. There could be safer cell phones and, yes, even safer wireless networks.

Building Biology experts W. Maes and F. Mehlis have raised this vital question in *Wireless Network, A Flyer by the Building Biology Association (VB), 2009:*

> Why are such antennas not activated except when they are actually needed, e.g. for the short period of time during a data transfer, and then automatically deactivated as soon as not in use? This would have been easy to accomplish, but the technical developers did not consider the possibility. An automatic deactivation was deliberately shortchanged.

Other Ways to Reduce Our EMR Exposure?

 With so many of our younger generation using mobile phones, wouldn't it be comforting to think that there was a quick and easy solution to protect them from the radiation? At this point, there does not seem to be a scientifically sound way to prevent all harmful biological effects with 'protective' devices.

Chips, Pendants etc.

People often ask me about the numerous devices on the market, such as radiation-deflecting/harmonizing chips that you stick on your cell phone or laptop, or about jewelry – pendants or bracelets – that you wear. These kinds of interventions are described as enhancing your own energy field in some way, and/or harmonizing/neutralizing the artificial electro-magnetic fields.

Some of these products seem to be helpful, for some people, at least for a while; many do not. I tried some of these myself, at one time. This technology, while promising, does not seem to provide the answer, just yet. Before investing, and trusting in this protection, you need to see some solid science on their effectiveness – not just testimonials. And insist on seeing the scientific evidence of how long the reported protection lasts.

And some clinicians advise that for some electro-sensitive people, these kind of protective interventions are contra-indicated because they may make symptoms worse.

The safety consultants I've talked with are concerned that 'magic bullets' like chips and pendants may lull people into a false sense of safety – they keep chatting away on their cell phones, keep their cordless phones and wireless router radiating day and night, believing they are now safe.

Seems more research is needed. Sensory Perspective in the UK has done an excellent service offering people the information and tools to protect themselves. The organization does not, however, recommend chips or other similar interventions.

One of their technical directors explains:

> Sensory Perspective focuses on what it knows will work: certifiably calibrated measuring instruments for detection, EMF barrier products for protection. We simply suggest that one uses suitable barrier products (shielded curtain materials, wallpapers, paints) for the home or office. www. detect-protect.com

Physical Radiation Barriers

These kinds of products are supposed to work by deflecting/blocking the radiation in some way. Stan Hartman comments on one example, pocket protectors: "I haven't tested any of them, but assuming that they shield the high frequencies from the phone, that still leaves the low-frequency magnetic fields from the battery-saver technology, which they can't shield.

It's best to just keep the phone at a distance in a purse or backpack or something – or toss it, of course. Certainly don't put it in a pocket over your heart."

Shielding Materials

If you've done everything you can to reduce your exposure, you may still want or need more protection from sources you can't control. In that case, you might have to do an EMR-repelling reno. This might include special window screens or films, wallpapers and EMR absorbing paints.

Stan Hartman gives us some expert advice on shielding:

> Keeping out microwaves is a little like trying to keep out blowing sand, though – you can do it, but you have to be sure there aren't any sources inside or any crevices for the radiation to get in through. That means no CFLs or other fluorescent lights, for instance, or CRTs – the old TV sets and computer monitors – or microwave ovens. If you have inescapable internal radiation sources, you could be better off not shielding at all and just trying to avoid radiation while you're sleeping at least, with a bed shield.

When it comes to shielding fabrics, wallpapers, paints, etc. caution is required. Shielding curtains, and bed canopies, are made from a fabric made of RF reflective fibers. This fabric is very effective at blocking RF – but you MUST use it properly, or you can get badly zapped! Some of these products have to be grounded. Do not use any of these without professional consultation, even if it's just a phone conversation with the supplier.

For example, the bed canopy fabric has to be properly draped away from the edges of the bed so it does not touch you, or any pet sleeping nearby. You cannot have any EMF/EMR sources inside the space draped by the fabric – no regular lamps, plugged in clocks, alarms etc.

So how do you read? A non-metal lamp, with an incandescent light bulb (not halogen or fluorescent) and shielded power cord is recommended.

And you need demand switches to reduce the electric and magnetic fields in the room before you use the fabric. A demand switch is a smart electronic device that automatically cuts off electricity when there is no demand for it. It also supplies electricity when there is a demand. Saves on your power bill, as well. This is one area where, unless you're a licensed electrician, you'll need professional help.

It's important to note that shielding devices, and therapeutic interventions, that may be very helpful for people without symptoms, can be devastating for electro-sensitive people, if not used properly.

At the end of the book, in Resources, I have listed sites in several countries, operated by qualified experts. You could begin your research there if you're considering adding these to your home.

Where to Start?

As you contemplate changes you might want to make in your family's technology habits, this thoughtful message from our "library mum" may be useful:

> As you know, my life is very hectic but I am now taking a break more often to get outside with the kids. It's great for them, and for me. I'm not even texting at the beach.
>
> And, thanks for Strategy 3, it was lucid, well set out and not frightening, after all. After reading it last night, I became convinced that it is necessary for us to have the discipline to do something about our cell phone use.
>
> We use the cell phones A LOT. Last night I proposed

that we get pagers. My husband disagreed, saying that if he is going to reduce the cell phone exposure, why would he replace it with exposure by some other gadget?

My cell phone is on today, but it is hidden in a location away from our house. It is on so that I can put it on call forwarding.

I will make a mental note to see if our server can do this automatically so that I don't have to have my cell phone on at all.

So, I see *Wireless Radiation Rescue* can be read on various levels. It can lead to basic changes – but it can also lead to quite profound changes. It has already instigated these more philosophical reflections on our life choices in our family.

Yes, Strategy 3 is packed full of cautions and recommendations. This can be quite a lot to take in, and more than you want to know?

I'd like to summarize some of them for you.

7 Key Reminders

Key point: choose wired over wireless, and corded over cordless

1. Switch your cordless phones to corded ones. Please don't give up your landline phone (and they are also health-savvy gifts);

2. Seek wired solutions for all things wireless, including your Internet access, keep laptops and all wireless devices off your lap, and please do not use digital baby monitors;

3. Keep your cell phone simple (basic, low SAR), and away from your head, your heart, pregnant women and the young. Limit it's use;

4. Use your mobile's speakerphone, rather than wireless, or wired headsets, and remember the most hazardous option of all is holding a mobile device against your head;

5. Avoid using a cell phone for an alarm, or sleeping near it;

6. Tell your airline and hotel that you want a wireless-free environment;

7. Talk to your local legislators, calmly and clearly. Provide some information (not overwhelming them) and ask for a response.

2 Minute Quick Read Summary

Strategy 4. Your Action Plan

Now that you understand – from Strategy 1 – why so many experts are concerned, and know how to recognize the related symptoms and conditions – from Strategy 2 – and have learned what sources you need to address – in Strategy 3 – you are well-outfitted to draft your priorities here, then go to Strategy 4 for your Action Plan.

Strategy 4 includes a room by room EMR audit; medical information about preventing and treating many symptoms and conditions that can be related; details on biological dentistry, and more. There is also a section on the Safer-Tech Family.

First, you might want to try this.

Our Radiation Rescue Intentions
Top Priorities - what I want to tackle first:

_____

Secondary priorities – what I want to deal with after that:

_____

I should consult a professional to assess the following:

_____

Other environmental exposures I want to address:

_____

See Strategy 4 for more details.

Strategy 4. Your Action Plan

Is anyone in your family already experiencing a lot of possibly related symptoms – difficulty sleeping, dizziness? Or one of the conditions that may be connected – headaches, insomnia, learning disorders, autism/Asperger's etc.?

If so, you will want to approach this step more vigorously as these people are more vulnerable.

If no one is experiencing symptoms, it does not mean the radiation is not having biological effects. It does give you the opportunity to reduce your family's exposure and risk of these symptoms and conditions.

You will also want to keep in mind the factors like proximity, intensity, duration/frequency as you decide on your priorities for action.

Room by Room – EMR Audit and Recommendations

Fairly soon I decided not to bog down in guilt, resentment or denial. I became determined to rescue my family and sought help, as I have explained, from the best sources I could find. Now all of that is set out here for you. Keep in mind this is not a quick fix; it is a process that takes some time.

My family began with a professional assessment. I strongly urge you to do the same, particularly if you are considering shielding fabrics, or other interventions that can cause problems if not used or installed correctly.

In the case of retro-fitting your home, or anything to do with electrical wiring, or shielding technology, it's wise to consult with and hire qualified professionals. Some of these are listed in the Resources section.

Testing of Your Home, Office and School

The Do-It Yourself Assessment – consumer devices to measure EMR are very helpful, not only in your own environment – but also vital when traveling (see Resources). You must know the basics, however, about the instruments, and what you are testing, or you can make your situation worse, not better. Like my friend with the microwave oven.

The Professional Assessment – this is key, in my view. Here is what Rob Metzinger (RM) advises: "Before the proper solutions can be implemented the primary sources of the problem – internal and external – must be identified."

Testing of Electric Fields, Magnetic Fields and RF (radio-frequency) should be done with the most sensitive testing equipment available.

The professionals' recommendations should look something like this:

1. Devices/sources to remove, perhaps in an order of priority for your situation: the urgent first-to-go, and then remove as you can, etc.

2. Devices/sources to replace, and with what ....

3. Alterations in position, use of the devices/sources etc.

4. Protective Interventions – shielding fabric etc.

Once solutions have been put in place the site must be re-tested to verify the efficacy of the products. Periodically the site should be retested to ensure the interventions are still performing and that new sources of contamination have not arisen.

Some Tips on Having a Professional Assessment

Before you have the pros come in it is helpful to label your electrical control panel. Make sure the person turning the breakers on and off is wearing non-conductive gloves, and is <u>not</u> electro-sensitive.

Mark each light switch and wall socket (in pencil) with the circuit number, and the same number, obviously, on the control panel (in pen). The technicians will check this but it saves you money if you can get a head start on this step.

Then they will go room by room – and outside of the building – to test for the electric, magnetic and radio-frequency.

As we move along through your house, in the following section, I'll share some of the things I learned during our audit, and add the experts' recommendations for safer/less harmful alternatives in square brackets, like this [...]

EMR Testing Equipment

If you are using testing equipment before, or instead of, a professional assessment, please be very careful. Three things to keep in mind:

1. Do you know how to use the meter?

2. Is it reliable – good enough quality? Consumer models may not measure the high frequency of that device – your cordless phone, for example, and give you a false 'safe' reading.

3. Are you using it for the right exposure? For example, you need a RF (radio-frequency) meter to test the radiation from a microwave oven, cordless phone – the handset or base, cell phone, wirelessly-connected computer etc. Remember the middle window of the spectrum?

For electrical outlets, appliances, heating pads and other wired devices you need a Gauss meter. See the Resources Section for a list of meters. Refer to the Building Biology Guidelines in Strategy 1.

If you get readings much higher than those levels, I really encourage you to get a professional assessment done. This is crucial if someone in your family is ill, pregnant, very young or very old.

Refer to the Resources section for qualified EMR testing and remediation consultants.

Most electricians are not experienced in this specific work and may assure you "there's no problem, it's all to code and within government standards." This response is a good signal to look for someone trained in this area.

Front Porch

Let's start this house tour right at the front door step. First, is there a wireless home security system, or a wireless front door bell [hard-wired options]. Is the front porch light fluorescent [low wattage incandescent]. An automatic garage door opener communicates wirelessly but is not considered a significant risk. [Just be mindful of this and don't point the clicker directly at anyone standing between it and the door. Same recommendation for the TV channel changer.]

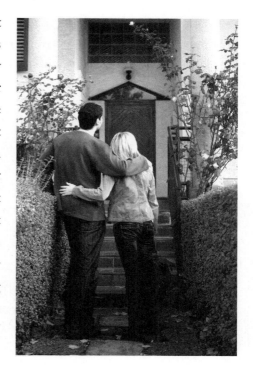

Bedrooms

The sleep zone is crucial to your wellbeing. As you may remember, EMR is known to disrupt sleep in many ways. Is your bedroom a radiation hot spot, or a calm low-tech oasis?

Besides looking at your own sleeping area, check out the places where children and/or pets sleep.

You are looking for: everything wireless, everything electric – all things plugged in – including clocks, radios, portable phones, TVs, electric beds, heaters, heating pads, electric cords, battery chargers, wall sockets, fluorescent (including compact fluorescent) or low voltage halogen lights, dimmer switches, lamps with transformers or the clap-on, or touch-on feature, everything metal – lamps, bed frames, headboard, footboard, side rails and box spring mattresses. No, you don't need to toss all of these, just note them and identify the ones that are creating high EMR.

[To reduce your EMR exposure, remove or unplug electronic devices located in the sleeping areas such as: televisions, DVD/VCRs, electric clock radios/alarm clocks, stereo systems, heating pads, electric blankets, and waterbeds. Battery-operated alarm clocks are a good alternative, or at least put the electric one a minimum of six feet away from your head.]

[If you absolutely have to have a television or a computer – with hard-wired Internet – in your bedroom, put them as far away as possible from the bed, and put them on a power bar that you turn off at night – or on a timer power bar.]

[Replace an electric blanket or heating pad with a hot water bottle or gel pack, or use the electrical kind just to heat up your bed, then turn off and unplug the cord before you get in.]

Metal is not recommended in sleeping areas as it reflects, and re-radiates, radiation from all surrounding sources, worsening exposures. Like most of us, you probably need to budget for many changes here. Science tells us that children are at least ten times more vulnerable to any toxic exposure than adults, so they need more protection.

[Making our children's bedrooms a priority, our technical experts urge us to: replace box springs with ones that contain no metal; replace coil and spring mattresses with foam mattresses made from low emission natural latex, or cotton mattresses such as futons (and to use natural cotton fabrics wherever possible to reduce static electricity); and to replace metal bed frames, metal cribs, metal bedside tables and lamps, metal bunk beds – with safer non-metallic types.]

[As we could afford it, I replaced these items, and our metal-framed bed with a solid wood one that even has wooden slats to hold the natural fiber futon mattresses.]

[My husband and I built a wooden reading lamp with a specially insulated electrical cord. We removed the halogen lamps with the transformers that had set the detector screaming.

And we replaced all fluorescent lights with regular incandescent ones.] Everyone in our family is mindful of energy consumption and we have many other ways to conserve energy and costs.

Ideally, and especially if you are suffering from any symptoms, shut off power in the rooms where you sleep and all the adjacent rooms, above and below this area, at night. This can be done by turning off the corresponding breakers, or by using a demand switch.

You may find inspiration in creating a low-tech, low EMR sanctuary where you sleep. Instead of a TV area, why not think about a space for calming practices like meditation, yoga or tai chi?

These have many benefits including balancing our life force energies that are so disrupted by electro-pollution – more on this later.

Children's Room

You want to go through your children's room with a sharp eye of awareness. Check for everything that is plugged in, the lights, electronic equipment etc. [Move the beds/cribs away from the wall – from any wall sockets and even the wiring in the wall. Avoid the use of sensor pads under baby.]

I'm presuming you are onboard by now in removing everything that hints of wireless – Internet access, cordless phones, wireless baby monitors [replace with low-powered plug-in ones, if you must have one].

[Use wooden beds without metal box springs or metal coiled mattresses. Use incandescent lights and battery alarm clocks.] Remember what Alasdair Philips told us about night lights – it's best to sleep in as dark a room as possible and that [plug-in red or orange, soft glow ones are preferred over white or blue lights, if we must have one.]

You might discuss this safer-tech reno with your children before yanking out their electronic entertainments and explain why you want their bedrooms healthier and safer for them. As you know, these issues are not high on any child's priority list.

Bathroom

You might test the electric toothbrush, electric razor and the hair dryer – using a Gauss meter. And check for microwave radiation around any mirrors or windows using a RF meter.

I realized the electric in-floor heating was not a great idea. Turning the dial down to "off" is not enough. [I had it disconnected.] Is the floor colder in the winter? Yes. But with a thick, cotton bath mat, it's fine. Also during that reno, I had found a quite large mirrored wall unit that we hung above the sink. It seemed like a great idea at the time. When the radiation detector "ghost busters" did our home assessment, the radiation bouncing off that mirror and metal cabinet was extreme.

(We may have to rethink some Feng Shui principles; while mirrors are considered good reflectors of energy, they do however also reflect what we could call the "negative energy" of EMR). [Now we have a small wooden framed mirror, and a small wooden shelf on the side wall.] After this EMR-busting retrofit, the radiation levels in the bathroom are now minimal.

As we've discussed, the health hazards in our homes are not all from EMR. Plastic shower curtains were found to off-gas toxic chemicals – and were still off-gassing a month after the package was opened! [I also replaced the plastic shower curtain with a fabric one.] And you may know about the chlorine and other chemicals in our tap water. [We have a filter on our shower head and another in the kitchen for our drinking and cooking water.]

You have the option of chemically- scented personal care products, cosmetics etc. [or the less toxic alternatives]. I discovered that virtually all standard brands of deodorant contain aluminum. Just 'trace amounts'. [All brands in natural health food stores are labeled "aluminum free".

Same recommendation goes for baby powder and baking powder – check for aluminum-free brands.] Dousing a newborn with sweet-smelling powder laced with aluminum? What are we thinking?

A friend reports on her home testing

On the weekend I used the device that measures wireless radiation. The three "hot spots" were the portable phone, cell phone and the wireless router near the kitchen.

The biggest shock came when I measured the microwaves coming from our portable phone. I had been happily using it as an alternative to my cell phone – thinking that my exposure would be less. In fact, the readings from the portable phone were 10 percent higher. The take away message for me is to get a corded landline.

I was also surprised to find the elevated readings from my cell phone when it was on standby. Suffice it to say, I am no longer using it as an alarm clock.

We have switched back to hard-wired Internet, as you suggested, and made the bedroom a low-electronic environment. Everyone seems to feel better – and sleep better. Thought it was just the stress.

Kitchen

Adults without health problems are fine in most kitchens, as long as they stand far away from microwave ovens when they are on. Those who should use more caution include: pregnant women, children, people with poor immune systems, convalescents, women with a history of breast cancer and men with a family history of testicular or prostate cancer.

When you're in the kitchen, you're often in the soup – of EMR. Test all plugged in appliances with a Gauss meter (microwave ovens also need testing with the RF meter, as you may remember). If you're shopping for new appliances, take the testing equipment to help you choose the best options.

How many counter-top gadgets do you have? [When I use the kettle or blender I stand back and unplug them when I've finished].

[When my fridge expired I replaced it with a no frills low energy consumption model. Each extra option that requires more power is going to increase the electro-magnetic field.

I also removed the under-the-counter CD player/radio that was only a few feet from my head when I was in the kitchen. Low intensity but high proximity and duration. The same player placed on the other side of the kitchen is no longer a concern].

The dishwasher, as you know, uses lots of energy and water, so being concerned about these, we don't run it more than we have to, always use the quick wash/air dry cycle, and don't stand against it when it's on.

In our kitchen there's no microwave oven, [reheating food on the stove only takes a few minutes]. What kind of stove do you have?

[Whenever possible I cook on the back burners on the stove as the electro-magnetic field from the front burners is much higher. The next time I buy a stove, I will get a gas stove and make sure it is well vented].

Gas stoves do not pose an EMR hazard as they don't use electricity. The sparks used to light the gas produce short bursts of high-voltage electricity, but these are insignificant. Some people with multiple chemical sensitivity need to avoid gas fumes.

Ovens, including fan-assisted convection ovens, electric fans/vents, even smaller toaster ovens are generating strong fields.

If you are standing close to the stove, with the front burners blasting, and the over-the-stove fan is on at your head, you are in a fairly strong field - test with a Gauss meter.

[Again the recommendation is stand back. Proximity is one of the best guidelines to keep in mind.]

Laundry Room

The same is true in the laundry room. Washing machines and dryers create strong electro-magnetic fields so it is best not to stand right beside them when they are on.

The other issue here is the toxic content of most laundry products unless they are one of the non-toxic natural brands. I once felt like leaving a Pilates class because most women had either washed their clothes in the standard detergent – chemically perfumed – or dried them with scented anti-static dryer sheets. I wanted to tell them that the chemicals from these products are absorbed through our skin. Ever walk past a house where people use these? You can detect the smell from the dryer exhaust.

Vacuum Cleaners

Most vacuum cleaners have powerful motors and give off high EMR. Strap-to-your-back kinds are *not* recommended. If you are pregnant, upright models are also not recommended. [The canister kind is preferred as the motor is further away from your body than upright models. Use a plain mop or broom for non-carpeted floors. Best not to use chemically-treated floor cleaning pads.]

Office

Whether we're talking about your home office, study, den or even your professional office, the same basic approach applies. We worked with the strongest exposures first – cordless and cell phones, other wireless devices, wireless Internet access and lighting. Then we tackled anything wired.

Your Cordless Phone Audit

How many cordless phones are in your home and office? Are they analog or digital? [We replaced all of ours with corded landlines that don't require electrical plugs, and use small batteries for the caller ID and speakerphone features.

You can also replace the handset cord with a 25 foot one, for long range wandering.]

Wireless Routers

Proximity is a factor, even with a long-range device such as this. [Every EMR expert strongly recommends replacing wireless Internet with a hard-wired system.

You might check out the kind that connects your Ethernet through the house wiring; you can plug into an electrical outlet for your Internet access. Not inexpensive, but has its benefits in reducing significantly your EMR exposure by taking wireless Internet out of your home.

If you must have a wireless router, place it as far away from sentient beings as possible, only power it on when you use it, and turn it off after that; always have it powered off at night.]

The radiation range from the average router is about 175 metres, (575 feet). At night, and when you're away, be considerate of your neighbors and switch it off. Any bees and other migrating beings whose natural navigation systems are being thrown out of whack will also be grateful.

It is recommended to stand back from all office equipment, printers, copiers, fax machines etc, when they are working.

And I won't mention another word about the microwave oven.

Experts' Action Plans

Many of these points have been touched on in previous sections, but it's interesting – and inspiring – to see how the leading authorities are putting their EMR-reduction advice into practice in their own homes and work places.

Dr. Martin Blank has no cell phone. His wife takes one in the car in case of an emergency. He has replaced his cordless phones with corded landlines. He's moved the electric clock away from the bed, got rid of circuits that have multiple electric switches on one line, as well as dimmer switches and instant-on devices.

He has also got rid of fluorescent bulbs in his house because they give off too much RF noise that has been linked to an increased risk of cancer.

Dr. Blank has meters and measures EMF levels at home from time to time. Instead of wireless Internet, Dr. Blank has a cable linkup between computers that are on opposite ends of the house. He and his wife do not own a microwave oven.

Dr. Hans Scheiner and his wife have had to make changes to their house because of their exposure to EMF from the proliferation of antennas in their area.

Testing with meters found the levels were very high in Dr. Scheiner's main floor medical clinic and in the 3rd floor bedroom. He has had the clinic walls coated with a special paint with small particles of carbon in it.

In the bedroom, the Scheiners have curtains made of shielding fabric, and on the outside wall have installed a thin metal plate that attracts electro-magnetic frequencies and grounds this energy into the earth. "The levels are much lower now."

Dr. William Rea offers his strategy for protecting his family from toxic exposures: "No cordless phones; no fluorescent lights, keep the chemical load down, consume organic food and safe water."

Rob Metzinger tells us:

"First, using special meters I evaluated exposure for Electric Fields, Magnetic Fields and RF (radio-frequency from microwaves – neighbors' cordless phones, wireless networks etc.) in all areas of the home, concentrating on the sleeping areas. Turned off power in all sleeping areas reducing electric field exposure by using demand switches.

• Removed all electronics from the sleeping areas.

• Installed shielded power cords on all computers and electronics.

• Moved computers and monitors as far away as possible from the users.

• Moved air conditioner away from children's sleeping area.

• Installed shielding curtains to deflect high levels of RF from entering the home.

• Replaced low voltage halogen, fluorescent and compact fluorescent lights with incandescent bulbs.

• Replaced dimmer switches with regular on/off switches

- Replaced spring mattresses with natural latex foam mattresses.

- Replaced electric alarm clocks with battery-operated units.

- Made a battery-operated night light for my children's rooms.

- Installed one analog 900 MHz cordless phone. All the other phones in our home are now land lines.

- Periodically retest exposure levels throughout the home.

- When purchasing any new electronic devices, I test them for EMF/ EMR emissions."

Action Plan – Environmental Health Factors to Consider

Because we can't control everything around us, even the best action plan, up to this point, is reducing our chemical and electrical exposures, but not eliminating them entirely.

At the end of this section, you will see the detailed Action Plan to fill out, if this is what you want to do.

You or someone you know may already have some of the EMR-related symptoms and conditions listed in the questionnaire in Strategy 2. Even if you haven't, you'll benefit from the recommendations from some eminent complementary health practitioners on how to protect and improve your health in this hyper-tech world.

First, have you ever wondered how the health of people in our advantaged society got so far off course? Let's take a look at how this might happen. This analogy of a river gives us insights into our own health challenges, and wellbeing strategies.

The River of Health – Pristine or Polluted?

The River Runs Clear

The clear mountain stream flows unhindered – translucent, its foundation bed of smooth river rocks can easily be seen. Light sparkles on its pristine surface and if you were to drink this pure, oxygen-rich water it would taste fresh and almost alive.

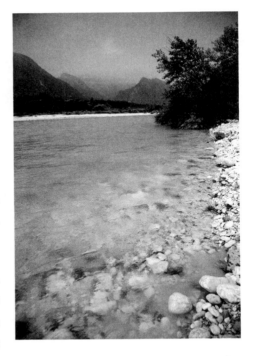

It is mineral rich, being fed by pure mountain streams, so its acid alkaline balance is as nature intended. The rocks over which it travels are free of debris. There are no blockages in the river; it is not twisted and its flow is not blocked. The river banks are clean and free of clutter.

Then at some point toxic sludge enters the river – at first this is absorbed by the river, diluted and purified.

Then at another place downstream, more sludge is introduced and bit-by-bit the river's ability to absorb and detoxify these toxins becomes compromised.

The once-clear waters become clouded; the river bed covered with a dark slime. Debris builds up on the river bank and the river narrows. In places, the river slows to a congested trickle. Problems arise at that blockage.

The flow of energy, blood and lymphatic fluid that sustain our health, and our lives, is much the same. Its path, twists and turns are partly set by our genetic heritage and family health history, but everything that enters it has an effect.

Ideally, we want to start our lives with as clean and strong a river of health as possible, but this is an increasing challenge in the modern world.

The average North American diet contributes a great deal of sludge to the river of life, including highly acidic foods (disrupting the pH balance), pesticides and herbicides, assorted additives and trans fats.

And emotional and/or physical traumas early in life also take a long-term toll on the body's ability to heal itself.

The River Reacts

Most children consume vast amounts of sugar and packaged foods – weakening the immune system and leaving them vulnerable to infection. Some children get recurring infections and lots of antibiotics. This can become a worrying cycle.

Antibiotics are truly wonder drugs and can save lives. Even if the family physician is careful only to prescribe antibiotics when strictly necessary, children may be ingesting antibiotics from foods such as industrially-raised chicken.

Antibiotics kill the bacteria we don't want, as well as wipe out the friendly bacteria – intestinal flora – that we need to maintain a healthy balance. A yeast overgrowth can result, overloading the immune system, leaving us vulnerable to more infections. If we are hit with a 'superbug' we may have nothing effective left in the arsenal.

Chemical sensitivities, asthma, even childhood cancers can arise from a compromised immune system, many experts advise. Systems are further burdened with mercury from vaccines and dental fillings.

The typical teenage diet of sugar, soda, fries, pizza and other fast foods is highly acidic. And many young people don't get enough sleep.

We have now set the ground for the potential of a lifetime of illness and disease. Later on in this section we'll look at a number of factors that combine to support our overall health. We can turn this around.

First, we'll start with electro-sensitivity, since this is a new condition, and most people – even many doctors – are not aware of how this exposure affects every system in our bodies.

Electro-hypersensitivity (EHS) – a new medical condition

We have a syndrome evolving called electro-sensitivity (ES), or electro-hypersensitivity (EHS). This is a phenomenon in which individuals experience recurring health effects which flare up while, or just after, they are exposed to electro-magnetic radiation.

As Dr. Magda Havas points out, there are heavily-radiated parts of the world where 3% of the population is so severely affected they have to live as far as possible from exposure. And she reports that as many as 35% have symptoms that significantly impair their quality of life.

In Sweden, EHS is officially recognized as a disability, so employers and building owners are expected to try to rectify the problems and sufferers may be entitled to disability benefits. While EHS is not an accepted medical diagnosis yet, the Canadian Human Rights Commission recognizes it as an environmental sensitivity and classes it as a disability.

Dr. Scheiner has treated thousands of people with EHS symptoms and agrees the number of people affected is on the rise:

> Some people are electro-allergic — not only sensitive but hyper-sensitive. When they are exposed they have headaches, sleeping problems, exhaustion during the day, dizziness, vomiting, tachycardia, concentration and memory problems. They may faint or their vision might be impaired. It's likely these are signs of opening of the blood-brain barrier. Doctors often tell them their symptoms are psychological.

Dr. Scheiner says an electro-hypersensitive person can usually recover from the symptoms by avoiding the exposure. The next step along the continuum is what he calls an electro-allergic reaction, in which the body's response is a real illness. Some will feel no ill effects — then suddenly will be hit with something as serious as cancer, high blood pressure or a stroke.

Thomas M. Rau, MD, the Medical Director of the Paracelsus Clinic in Lustmühle, Switzerland, is convinced electro-magnetic loads lead to cancer, concentration problems, ADD, tinnitus, migraines, insomnia, arrhythmia, Parkinson's Disease and even back pain:

> At the Paracelsus Clinic (www.paracelsus.ch), cancer patients are now routinely educated in electromagnetic field remediation strategies, and inspectors from the Geopathological Institute of Switzerland are sent to patients' homes to assess electro-magnetic field exposures.

Source: www.electromagnetichealth.org, 'Electromagnetic Load a Hidden Factor in Many Illnesses' February 2009.

Medical Help on the Horizon for People with EHS

In June of 2010, Dr. Heather McKinney attended the American Environmental Health Foundation (AEHF) and the University of North Texas Health Science Center conference in Dallas. The focus was on the Chemical Mechanisms Leading to EMF (electro-magnetic field) Sensitivity. If you are dealing with chemical and/or electro-sensitivity, you will be heartened to hear about this gathering, and the progress in diagnosing and treating this, and related, conditions.

Dr. McKinney offers this to us:

> Physicians, researchers, scientists, nutritionists, counselors, and patients met to better understand and address the physiological signs and symptoms of electro-sensitivity. Their summary: the body is an electrical system that acts as an antenna — absorbing and receiving various information and sensations, including electro-magnetic fields from wired and wireless technologies.
>
> Health professionals from Australia, Brazil, Canada, Japan, the UK, and the USA discussed emerging ideas for testing, triggers, signs/symptoms, treatments and resources. Here are some of the highlights:
>
> **Testing strategies**: heart rate variability, blood sugar, live blood analysis, heavy metal test/hair analysis, mold/allergy testing, and lymphocyte sensitivity.
>
> **Triggers**: environmental and chemical stress, mold, thermal changes (exposure to heat/cold), sun spots, certain foods.

Signs and Symptoms: poor circulation, skin changes, tremors, migraines, seizures, rapid heartbeat, diabetes, MS, chronic fatigue, asthma, allergies, food sensitivities/intolerance, memory fog, Alzheimer's and autism.

Possible Treatments: decreasing exposure to EMF (wireless, electronics, compact fluorescent light bulbs), hydration – drinking lots of pure water, adrenal and immune support, vitamins/supplements including magnesium and Vitamins B, C and D, hormone support, removing mercury fillings (with strict controls), acupuncture, chiropractic and other energy therapies, meditation, yoga, deep breathing techniques, homeopathy, Epsom salt baths, rotation diet, medically-supervised chelation and decreased exposure to metals.

AEHF has created a forum for open dialogue among professionals and patients. The faculty panel praised efforts for education in the area of electro-sensitivity, including possible causes, treatment, relief, support, and further research. Education will help bridge the gap between science and healthcare professionals, and those experiencing this medical condition.

Perhaps the most promising take away message from the conference is the faculty panel's commitment to independent research and education. Personally, I was inspired by the commitment and expertise of the health professionals from around the world, and the dedication of the patients – not only to help themselves, but to inform others about this condition. There is, as Kerry Crofton writes, hope for the future.

No, EMR does not cause everything.

At this stage you may well be wondering how electro-magnetic radiation can be blamed for such a lengthy and diverse list of symptoms and conditions. According to data compiled by Paul Raymond Doyon, MA, research indicates "there are about eighty immune system disorders that we didn't have twenty-five years ago before we really started microwaving the planet." Is there a connection, one wonders?

Whether a person develops symptoms, or not, can be influenced by the intensity and duration of the exposure, and by the individual's vulnerability – whether his or her overall health and immunity are strong enough to buffer the effects of EMR.

Reportedly, that is why ES/EHS is more common in people who already have chemical, or other environmental, sensitivities. Many may also be burdened by heavy metals in their systems and by food allergies.

Dr. Scheiner also says people who have had cancer are more susceptible to developing electro-hypersensitivity; their bodies are likely too busy fighting the cancer to be able to fend off this extra assault.

Even when exposure to EMR hasn't directly caused a disease, for instance diabetes, or a neurological condition such as MS, ALS or Parkinson's, the medical experts tell us that the symptoms may get worse as the person's body tries to cope with the additional burden of this exposure.

EHS Symptoms and Related Conditions

(with the kind permission of Susan Parsons: www.weepinitiative.org)

SYMPTOMS OF ELECTRO HYPERSENSITIVITY					
Neurological		**Cardiac**	**Respiratory**	**Dermatological**	**Ophthalmologic**
headaches	depression	palpitations	sinusitis	skin rash	deteriorating vision
difficulty concentrating	anxiety	pain or pressure in the chest	asthma	facial flushing	pain or burning in the eyes
muscle and joint pain	confusion and spatial disorientation	low or high blood pressure	bronchitis	itching	pressure in/behind the eyes
memory loss	fatigue	shortness of breath	pneumonia	burning	floaters
dizziness	weakness	arrhythmia			cataracts
nausea	tremors	slow or fast heart rate		swelling of face and neck	
irritability	muscle spasms				
numbness	leg/foot pain				
tingling	"Flu-like" symptoms				
hyperactivity	fever				
altered reflexes	insomnia				
OTHER					
digestive problems	abdominal pain	testicular/ovarian pain/swelling	enlarged thyroid	great thirst	dehydration
nosebleeds	internal bleeding	hair loss	pain in the teeth	deteriorating fillings	Light sensitivity
swollen lymph nodes	loss of appetite	hypoxia	allergies	frequent urination and incontinence	night sweats
immune abnormalities	redistribution of metals within the body	ringing in the ears (tinnitus or similar chronic ear-noise)	impaired sense of smell	altered sugar metabolism	dryness of lips, tongue, mouth, eyes
Severe reactions can include seizures, paralysis, psychosis, and stroke					

Doesn't it seem incredible that just about everything you've ever heard of is here? How could this be? Medical experts I've talked with explain this by saying that EMR affects every cell, organ and system in the body. So if you consider this, it doesn't seem as hard to believe that there are so many related symptoms and conditions.

If your house were flooded repeatedly, eventually everything within it would be affected.

How can you tell whether your symptoms are EMR related, or not? This is just what I asked Dr. Scheiner. He explained that each symptom might be unspecific (in other words not related to a particular illness):

> You can have a headache for a lot of reasons. It gets specific if you get lots of them, or sleeping problems. If you can't sleep at night this could be microwave syndrome from EMR exposure... not yet a sickness, it's a warning syndrome.

> The body is saying 'I am having trouble here'. It is a call for help. Allergies and food sensitivities could also be a test.

More women than men? Not so.

Dr. Scheiner also makes a gender observation:

> Women seem to have a finer sensitivity to their symptoms and to heed them more. Often men who attend our clinic will say 'I have *no* problem, but my wife really suffers.' Then we do some lab tests and discover both are being biologically affected equally.

A short wilderness retreat, if away from cell antennas, can give you useful information. Dr. Scheiner suggests removing yourself from some of the sources for a few days, and seeing what happens. If the headaches, insomnia, tingling and other symptoms improve when you're away, and return when you come back, this is probably a sign that you're electro-sensitive.

Cindy Sage of the BioInitiative Group, agrees:

> Symptoms quickly improve when away from EMF/EMR sources, particularly when the patient moves away from computers, fluorescent lighting, transformers, wireless antenna, cell and cordless phones, appliances and out of proximity to cell phone towers, electrical substations and power lines...

> Symptoms recur on returning to the irradiated environment. Over time, sensitivity is increased to smaller and smaller EMF/EMR exposures.

The renowned surgeon Dr. William Rea, offers the EHC-D protocol used at his Environmental Health Center – Dallas (www.ehcd.com). This facility is a complete testing and medical treatment clinic for environmentally-sensitive adults and children.

1. Eliminate exposure
2. Energy balancing
3. Mineral analysis
4. Skin test for minerals
5. IV nutrients twice weekly
6. Grounding at least 1 hour/day
7. Immune modulation
8. Sauna

Katharina Gustavs says, "Grounding and sauna, as mentioned above, are great therapeutic strategies for healing. However, if the grounding involves artificial grounding pads, the electric field exposure could increase during the grounding. Walking barefoot along the beach, of course, is always a winner. Infrared saunas are notorious for high magnetic and electric field exposures."

One company that has been recommended has evidence that its low EMR emission infrared saunas are specifically designed for electro- and chemically-sensitive people. (See the Resources section.)

Sarah Dacre, a leading advocate in the UK, reports she has reduced her disabling EHS symptoms – with a variety of interventions:

> After a few years of dealing with this, I now have 95% of my perfect memory back. How did I achieve this? By shielding my life from EMR; moving my bed; switching off all EMF emitting devices and detoxifying. I drink only spring water and eat a very healthy home cooked diet, and take pure supplements and minerals.
>
> I sleep on a foam mattress supported by a wooden bed. I have regular Chinese acupuncture where the remedial focus is on memory and a healthy central nervous system.
>
> Additionally, I no longer use a mobile (cell) phone, which caused me withdrawal symptoms. I went through cold turkey from this addiction. My right eyesight has since improved enough not to wear glasses.
>
> I walk in nature every day both for the exercise and fresh air, oxygen is vital to assist my body cope with its heavy toxic load.

The WEEP Initiative has a section on living with EHS on its website, www.weepinitiative.org/livingwithEHS.html

Now, let's keep going and look at a few more conditions and explore how EMR exposure influences them. You may discover some connections with health issues in your family, and some useful medical advice.

Our library mum – a woman who has been reading parts of the book as they've been written – has noted some interesting inter-connections:

> It seems EMR is one of *various* environmental toxins that we are exposed to which are compromising our immune system. A couple of years back, I was exposing myself to a lot of bleach and when I stopped this, I recovered much of my health (slowly, over time). The challenge is that it is difficult to put our finger on *which* environmental toxin is the culprit because it is the overall load of toxins that get us...we need to abandon the search for a single cause.

Immune System Impairment

The Sweet Smell of...Chemical Overload?

Why should you care about this? We only have one immune system, one lymphatic system, one liver, one set of kidneys etc, to deal with the daily onslaught of environmental toxins, EMR now included.

Your immune system, whether you know or not, is reacting to all of these environmental exposures. The more we can reduce the various chemical loads, the better it is for us, and for all life forms on this planet, including the birds in the air, and the fish in the rivers and oceans.

And most people who are electro-sensitive are also chemically sensitive, so this is vital information for them.

I asked Dr. William Rea what is of most concern to him these days. His answer: "Pesticide exposure plus wireless equipment. EMF sensitivity is a growing problem in the world. Everyone needs to be aware of its consequences."

Dr. Rea elucidates on the interplay of environmental influences:

> Various factors (heavy metals, inner terrain – yeasts, pH balance, emotional stress etc.) may combine to make us more vulnerable to a myriad of environmental toxins, including EMR. Dealing effectively with these factors can boost our ability to buffer the toxic effects. If the load is reduced, many times the patient can tolerate the EMR.

Systems Overwhelmed?

A recent report on the rapid rise of serious food allergies in children (including life-threatening ones like peanuts) tells us that the experts cannot explain the nearly 20% increase in the last decade. Could it be the deluge of chemicals in our air, food and environment are overwhelming young immune systems?

Some companies were recently defending the several carcinogens found in their baby lotions and bath products, as just 'trace amounts'. I have also discovered one also needs to be vigilant for the wolf in sheep's clothing: chemically-laden products are labelled "natural" or "fresh", or some such disguise. A story comes to mind: when I had a counseling practice, a woman told me that she had used a plug-in air freshener for her son's bedroom to purify the air to help with his asthma. Like most of us, she was getting her health information from marketers.

You have probably heard that lead, tar and formaldehyde are used in most cosmetics and 'personal care products'. When they say 'perfume', unless they are using only essential oils, assume these are chemicals, as in most scented candles, cleaning products, air fresheners. Taking these things out of your home can ease everyone's immune and respiratory systems. Here's some more good information from Larry Gust:

> Fragrances commonly use phthalates, some of which are hormone disrupters. These, as well as synthetic musk compounds and other chemicals, accumulate in human tissue and are found in breast milk. Manufacturers don't necessarily test this stuff for neurological effects or respiratory effects — even though we know an increasing number of people have asthma attacks when exposed to scented products and two fragrance materials that had been used for decades were found to be neurotoxic.

Can we live in a pure, non-toxic environment? I don't think so. And, yes, our immune systems need a good workout — so we shouldn't swab down the decks too often with anti-bacterial soaps.

However, given the chemical pollutants in our environment it is wise to reduce all the exposures we can, and not agonize about the ones we cannot, and boost our ability to handle these — a serenity prayer for health. This will bring benefits as we age. Anti-aging experts advise a less polluted environment enhances health and longevity, as well as appearance. Reducing electro-pollution exposure is crucial. This new factor is missing in most anti-aging programs.

Dr. Mark Hyman is a physician who emphasizes the benefits of addressing environmental pollutants, including EMR:

> Clearly there are many environmental influences that can have a major impact on overall health, including your brain health. These toxins affect us all from our food, our water and air, medications, chemicals, metals, molds and electromagnetic radiation.
>
> Everyday choices we make to protect ourselves will have impact globally. The European Union, through new legislation (called REACH) designed to limit toxins in commercially produced goods, caused China to change its manufacturing practices.
>
> Buying organic food, refusing vaccines with mercury, or buying deodorant without aluminum will create a ripple effect throughout our economy and environment.
>
> You *can* heal yourself from brain damage by altering your diet, limiting your exposure to toxins, and changing the way you live. You can REVERSE the effects of depression, anxiety, bipolar disorder, autism, Alzheimer's, ADHD, and more if you know how to.
>
> From *The UltraMind Solution,* (Simon & Schuster 2009)

Chronic Fatigue Syndrome (CFS) In the UK, this condition is called myalgic encephalomyelitis (ME).

Several of our experts have advised us that EMR exposure weakens the immune system. An overwhelmed immune system cannot fend off environmental toxins, bacteria and viruses leaving us more open to colds, flu etc. Not only do we get sick more often, it can take us much longer to recover. And we feel more tired, more often.

A compromised immune system is also a contributing factor in, and a result of, Chronic Fatigue Syndrome, and many other conditions. (As you may know, emotional stress also weakens our immune systems.)

While CFS/ME is a complex illness with many possible causes, in October 2009 an American research team reported, in the journal *Science*, that a single retrovirus – a blood-borne pathogen – may play a major role. Retroviruses are known to cause neurological symptoms, cancer and immunological deficiencies, and many people with chronic fatigue report their symptoms emerged after a serious viral infection.

While it's too early to say whether this discovery will lead to better treatments, the news is heartening to the millions of people worldwide who suffer from this debilitating condition.

The reason I am including a section on this is that CFS and exposure to electro-magnetic radiation share many symptoms and are connected. And knowing about CFS can be a great boost to your overall health and your ability to heal from, or ward off, the effects of EMR.

In 1983, W. Grundler, in Germany, found even very low levels of EMR exposure affects the increased growth of yeast cells.

("Sharp Resonances in Yeast Growth Prove Nonthermal Sensitivity to Microwaves").

Dr. Rau adds his recommendations for dealing with electro-sensitivity and fighting yeast conditions:

> Cultures have shown beneficial bacteria grow more slowly in the presence of electromagnetic fields allowing pathological (yeast – candida) organisms to dominate. Thus, a strategy with electrically sensitive patients, or with those facing chronic conditions, is the aggressive

supplementation with probiotics and other Biological Medicine approaches to balance intestinal flora. Many people with chronic infections likely linked to EMR exposures, such as Lyme Disease, are symptom-free after an aggressive microorganism rebalancing program.

A proliferation of yeast cells (Candida albicans) in the bowel can be a contributing factor in many conditions, including Chronic Fatigue Syndrome, and will weaken the health of EHS people.

A physician specialising in complementary medicine, Carolyn Dean MD ND, author/coauthor of 17 books including *The Magnesium Miracle,* explained in a recent interview that it's not just fatigue:

> In brief, Candida albicans is a fungus living in our intestines that produces 180 chemical toxins capable of making you feel dizzy and fatigued, shutting down your thyroid, throwing your hormones off balance, and causing you to crave sugar and alcohol, and gain weight. It's associated with drowsiness, insomnia, numbness, tingling, PMS, loss of libido, painful intercourse, infertility, MS, Crohn's, colitis, IBS, acne, Lupus, white tongue, bad breath, body odor, sinusitis, bruising, sore throat, bronchitis, shortness of breath, heart palpitations, spots in front of eyes.

> The miracle of antibiotics has its downside as an underlying cause of yeast overgrowth. The refining of sugar and wheat has its downside by creating a simple food source for yeast.

> The tremendous levels of stress hormones that flood our bodies daily also make us prey to yeast. When yeast, bacterial, and food toxins hit the blood stream they

trigger widespread inflammatory reactions by either directly attacking tissues or creating allergic reactions along with the production of histamine. It is mainly through diet and lifestyle change that you can overcome yeast overgrowth—but you *can* overcome it, and reduce the amount of inflammation in your life with some effort and support.

Original article: Total Health and Longevity Magazine Sept 2006 issue.

Dr. Dean also describes how magnesium can be useful in CFS and possibly EHS as these conditions share many symptoms, including insomnia and fatigue, as we have seen:

> Magnesium-deficient patients commonly experience fatigue because dozens of enzyme systems are under-functioning. An early symptom of magnesium deficiency is fatigue.

Dr. Dean is the medical director of the Nutritional Magnesium Association and has a wellness consulting practice in Hawaii.

The treatment suggested for CFS, and boosting one's immune system, includes cutting out sugar. Sadly, the more difficult this is, the more it may be needed, as craving sweets is one of the main symptoms. Physicians specializing in this also recommend supplementing with good quality probiotics – it's not enough to eat yogurt – and using an effective anti-fungal. There are more details at Dr. Dean's website: www.drcarolyndean.com

Another physician specializing in complementary medicine, and an expert in CFS, Dr. Jacob Teitelbaum has more information on the treatment of CFS on his site www.endfatigue.com. I asked Dr. Teitelbaum this question: "Many people, including those with EMR exposure, are tired and don't sleep well. So how do you know if you really have CFS?"

> Although many people are tired and have poor sleep, the fatigue usually goes away with rest and is not associated with the other symptoms. It is the mix of a common group of symptoms that define a syndrome. People who are tired, achy, 'brain foggy', can't sleep, have increased thirst and poor libido – even if these are not disabling – often have a milder form of CFS.

Electro-sensitivity and CFS

Dr. Teitelbaum offers his responses to a patient experiencing sensitivity to electric fields and computers.

Q. "I had a relapse with CFS and have been out of work for a year. I notice that this time around a few months into the illness, that I am now sensitive to sitting in front of a computer screen. Symptoms: I feel hot and nauseated, and if I stay on the computer long enough, feel my heart racing. I notice that I'm really sensitive to it in the morning versus the evening. Any ideas?"

Dr T. "There are those who get electro-sensitivity with CFS. In some cases, turning off the electric circuit to your bedroom before you go to bed (use a wind up alarm clock or a battery one kept away from your head) and leaving the electricity off at night (you would be amazed at some of the electromagnetic fields found in the bedroom) can also help – especially since you report feeling worse in the morning.

In severe cases, there are specialists that can evaluate a home for electrical pollution and assist in remediation."

Sleep, perchance to dream?

The curtains are drawn tightly. The spacious room is dark and seemingly conducive to sleep. The woman in the brass bed has one arm twisted around the sheets; the other's flung out the side and rests lightly on her wireless laptop. On the night table the digital clock marks the minutes of another sleepless night.

Her trouble falling sleep, and then staying asleep, seems to be getting worse. "Stress, no doubt," the doctor advises and prescribes pharmaceuticals. Annoyingly, these seem to make her dozier during the day than they do at night. These pills perch on the table along with an arsenal of headache remedies. She read that room temperature is crucial, so, she either snuggles a heating pad, or relies on an air conditioner. Nothing is working.

Ever resourceful, she has surrounded herself with the latest techno-delights. In the middle of the night she often she flicks on the light and taps away on her laptop, or picks up her cell phone and calls a friend in an earlier time zone. She likes its all-in-one convenience – she can shop online, plan vacations, stay in touch, and the alarm is so pleasing she tucks it under her pillow. There's also a cordless phone on her night stand; being an early adopter she has the power-packed DECT 6.0 model, accessorized with a touch-screen for the ultimate in wireless chic. She no longer feels sleepy. Then, she looks over and sees the clock …

Insomnia, Stress, Mood

As you may know too well, not being able to sleep affects every facet of your life to the point where you can barely function. Specialists say it doesn't take long before sleep deprivation drives down your IQ (temporarily!), impairs reasoning and memory, makes adults more irritable and kids a little more "hyper".

As if that isn't enough, scientists also suspect that chronic sleep deprivation in children may also impair their growth and development. There are of course many factors that contribute to sleep disruption — caffeine, stress, hormones, a bedroom that faces a noisy street...

Not too long ago, our family was staying at a hotel when I attended a conference. I had chosen this hotel because it was one of the few that did not have wireless Internet access in the room.

My relief was short-lived, however, when I got into our room, looked out the window, and saw a nearby cell tower antenna. I had a small RF meter, which had a very sensitive audio signal. The levels were so high that this meter screamed as loud as it does next to a cell phone in use.

It wasn't easy explaining to the front desk why we wanted to change our room. I found a room on a lower floor, with less exposure, but when we left the hotel, I felt a pang of sadness for people seeking help in the sleep research centre that was on the top floor of this building. (Also I felt for the housekeeping staff with powerful vacuum cleaners strapped to their backs. Intensity. Proximity. Duration.)

In stress disorders and depression, EMR has been shown to affect levels of brain chemicals and hormones including norepinephrine, dopamine and serotonin, which are involved in regulating mood.

As you may know, these conditions are already epidemic so more research is needed here. Maybe this why we feel more calm, and our spirits are lifted, when we are out in nature and far removed from technology.

As Dr. Scheiner describes, your ability to sleep can be a good indicator of your EMR exposure and sensitivity.

Many people who are not sleeping well may be unknowingly immersed in a high EMR environment. We know the agitating effect of EMR on the brain. Is it any wonder that difficulty sleeping is one of the primary and most prevalent symptoms?

Evidently, some people are using electric mattress pads to sleep better, and/or to enhance their health. You may remember reading about why this is a problem, in Strategy 3.

EMR exposure has been shown to make it more difficult to "wind down" and can also reduce the amount of melatonin in the brain. According to some research, using a cell phone for more than 25 minutes a day for two weeks can be enough to reduce melatonin levels. Katharina Gustavs adds, "According to J. Burch's research, the effect is exacerbated if you sit in a dimly lit office for most of the day."

As you may know, this hormone is necessary for deep, restful sleep, which also allows the body to recharge and heal itself.

(Many years ago, a remarkable immunologist told me that one of the primary functions of sleep was to recharge the immune system.)

A small study done by Sweden's Karolinska Institute and Uppsala University, with Wayne State University in Detroit, released in January 2008, revealed that people using a cellphone just before bedtime took longer to get into deep sleep, and spent less time in this deeper sleep phase.

(Published by the Massachusetts Institute of Technology's Progress in Electromagnetics Research Symposium).

One of the researchers, Dr. Bengt Arnetz, said it appears that cell phones affect the areas of the brain responsible for activating and co-ordinating the stress system. It's also possible that radio waves disrupt production of melatonin, which controls the body's internal circadian rhythms.

Melatonin performs many crucial functions including regulating the timing of the onset of puberty.

Therefore it's no wonder sleep experts such as Dr. Jeffrey Lipsitz were especially disturbed by what this study implies for teenagers, who tend to use cell phones more in the evening, talk for long periods of time, and keep the phones on standby during the night.

As he told CTV News, a Canadian TV network:

> If they're using cell phones for long hours in the evening and then going to sleep and their sleep is disturbed this may have implications with regard to health and development and functioning in school and so on...

Insufficient sleep in young people is linked to mood and personality changes, ADHD-like symptoms, depression, lack of concentration and poor academic performance.

Dr. Lipsitz went on to say:

> You kind of wonder what else might be going on to the brain as a result of extended cell phone use, and what does that mean for all of us?... It certainly cries out for more research.

(Incidentally, the study was funded by the Mobile Manufacturers Forum, which called the results "inconclusive.")

Dr. Jacob Teitelbaum also writes about insomnia in *From Fatigued to Fantastic* and recommends: "magnesium 75 to 250 mg and calcium, 600 mg at bedtime and Hydroxy L-tryptophan (5-HTP) 200 to 400 mg at night. 5-HTP is what your body uses to make serotonin, a neurotransmitter that helps improve the quality of sleep." It may take four to six weeks to see the full effect of 5-HTP, though, so don't expect instant results.

Dr. Teitelbaum cautions that if you're taking anything else that raises your serotonin levels (including SSRI-type anti-depressants or even herbal remedies like St. John's Wort), "it is reasonable to limit the 5-HTP to 200 mg at night." In rare cases people may experience a reaction from excess serotonin.

As with all supplements that affect the body's natural production of hormones, for example, you should consult with a qualified clinician – physician or naturopathic doctor – before following any protocols. There may be contra-indications, conflicts with certain conditions and/or medications you need to know about.

Dr. Teitelbaum also has some useful insight:

> For most people with disordered sleep, supplementing melatonin to normal levels takes 3/10ths of a milligram. The usual dose is 3 milligrams, which is ten times the level I recommend.

I have found that sleeping in a dark room, and one that stays dark until you want to wake up, is very helpful. Try blackout curtains, or good eyeshades. Did you know that eyeshades keep the light out of your eyes and help in sleeping, but you need the whole room darkened to enhance the production of sleep-inducing melatonin? And, of course, make your bedroom a low EMR sanctuary.

Sleeping Well Beyond the Electronic Cocoon

This once-sleepless mom heard our alert – loud and clear – and took action right away:

> I am a recovering breast cancer patient, and a life long skeptic, but after reading this book I found the information in the book so compelling, that I decided to make some immediate changes.
>
> To start, I replaced my cordless phones with land lines, moved my blackberry charger out of my bedroom, moved my bedside clock across the room, and stopped sleeping with the blackberry on my night table. We removed all of my daughter's electronics from her room, and got rid of her metal bed frame. As a family, we decided to try out a self-imposed one-hour-per-day-limit on how much time we would spend in front of the computer, television, DS and Wii for a month, and see what happened. We recognized

that there may have to be adjustments to computer time made to manage work and/or school obligations. To be honest, while it seemed like the right thing to do, I didn't expect to notice any immediate effect. However, I have been struggling with insomnia for the past three years, two years prior to my breast cancer diagnosis. The first night after clearing all of the electronics out of my room, I slept like a baby. Likewise for the next night.

While I am willing to consider a certain amount of placebo effect, I have now been sleeping well and deeply for a few weeks. I notice that I rarely wake in the night to use the washroom (before, I would get up several times in the night) and when I do wake up, I fall easily back to sleep.

My daughter, who at 13 has been complaining about not sleeping well for the last year, is also sleeping more deeply. Now that I think about it her sleeping difficulties began about the same time we put a cordless phone in her room, and mine began when I got my blackberry. Maybe just two coincidences. Or maybe not.

During my period of sleeplessness, I stopped drinking caffeine, and did everything I could to improve the quality of my sleep. I looked at all of the possible causes - new job, peri-menopause, caffeine intolerance, food allergies. I worked with a naturopath. While there was some small improvement, nothing was as dramatic as the effect of lowering the EMR levels in my bedroom and house.

My son has ADD and learning disabilities, and we wonder what other benefits our experiment in "unplugging" will reveal. Last night, we went to the park and played tennis after school, then had a rousing game of UNO after dinner. Playing cards and tennis are much preferable to the poor habits we had been slipping into, with each of us isolated in our individual electronic cocoons.

Cardiovascular – Heart disease, TIA, Stroke

Cardiovascular disease is a major problem in industrialized countries, and it's not just because of the unhealthy western diet. Researchers explain that when EMR depletes the levels of antioxidants in the blood, high-density lipoproteins (HDL), the good cholesterol, will bind with free radicals (oxidants) turning the good cholesterol into bad cholesterol (LDL). This leads to thicker, "stickier" blood, which can form clots. (Emotional stress also thickens the blood, and constricts the arteries.)

And EMR has been shown to disturb our own sensitive electrical system – the brain and the heart, for example.

I have a friend who is a scientist at a leading university. Despite being fit, and in otherwise excellent health, she was rushed to emergency in cardiac distress. There's a claim by staff that a cluster of cancers is related to the high levels of EMR on her campus.

Could the cardiac symptoms also be related? Some electro-sensitive people can actually tell when there is a cell phone powered on nearby – they feel a change in their heart rate and rhythm, and/or a tightness in their chest.

Years ago I co-produced a program for Canadian network TV on heart health. I'd like to reconnect with the hundreds of patients I counseled when I worked in cardiac clinics, and encourage them to read this research and do an EMR audit of their homes and workplaces.

And I'd like to go back to all the cardiologists I once knew to ask if they're seeing an increase in "unexplained" cardiac symptoms.

In November 2009, Dr. Havas presented research demonstrating increased heart rate from wireless radiation exposure. Evidence included an increase in heart rate on exposure to a nearby cordless phone. The heart rate immediately returned to the baseline after that phone was unplugged (see www.magdahavas.com).

There is a concern that many patients today who are experiencing cardiac, and other electro-hypersensitivity, symptoms are turning to prescription drugs, instead of reducing their EMR exposure.

I welcomed this pioneering study and the opportunity to ask cardiologist Dr. Stephen Sinatra for his insight. He told me that he applauded Dr. Havas's research and offered this observation:

> We saw these cardiac effects ourselves in the middle of a study when a cordless phone was in use. If electro-pollution stresses the body like emotional stress then we already have mountains of evidence on how this affects our health including, of course, the cardiovascular system.

Ophthalmological/Vision Problems

EMR has been shown to damage the lens of the eye. According to Powerwatch, this has been known for more than forty years:

> In 1964 Dr. Milton Zaret was one of the first scientists to speak out about the dangers of microwave radiation and ocular effects. According to Zaret, exposure to this radiation at either thermal, or non-thermal, levels can cause cataracts which sometimes remain latent for months or years. Zaret then had his laboratory research funds cut off.

Metal eyeglasses can attract EMR, magnifying its effects. (Here's another tip from an eye surgeon: blue-tinted lenses are not recommended as they let in harmful rays of the light spectrum.) Another expert has told me that our eyes are one of the tissues that are especially endangered by exposure to EMR. The other particularly vulnerable body parts are the testicles.

Infertility, Miscarriages, Birth Defects

For couples longing to conceive, all this is deeply distressing. Some researchers in human reproduction are now telling us the more time men spend on cell phones, or carry powered-on phones in the pockets of their pants, the lower their sperm quality.

Other work exposure to EMR may also be a factor in men's reduced fertility. A study of 17 thousand military employees in the Norwegian navy, between 1950 and 2002, found men who worked within ten miles of high frequency aerials had a significantly higher risk of infertility than the ones who worked farther away. (Baste V, Riise T, Moen BE Eur J Epidemiol 2008)

In Japan, with its massive concentration of electro-smog, an unusually high number of women are suffering miscarriages in their last trimester. (Nagaishi et. al., J.*Obstet Gynaecol Res.* 2004)

In August 2009, Dr. Louis Slesin of Microwave news reported:

> Martine Hours, the chief science advisor to the French RF research program, has called for serious studies on the effects of cell phones on male fertility. Now, Australia's John Aitken is saying the issue 'deserves our immediate attention.' In a new study, Aitken has reported that cell phone radiation damages human sperm – as well as DNA. Cell phone use and radiation has now been shown to harm sperm, in five different countries and including two different groups in the United States, one of which is at the Cleveland Clinic. Aitken's message is simple: Men who want to have children should not keep active mobile phones in their trouser pockets.

When couples trying to conceive know that EMR exposure decreases fertility they can now make informed decisions.

More girls than boys in your play group?

There are also indications of a global prevalence of female births. Some researchers suspect this may be due to EMR. A Russian study in the 1950's found an altered sex ratio (more girls) in children born during the years of a radar station's operation in what was known as Latvia. That Norwegian navy study, which I mentioned above, showed similar results: a lower ratio of boys to girls were born to fathers who reported a higher degree of exposure to high-frequency antennas and communication equipment.

Evidently, the normal sex ratio is commonly 105 boys to 100 girls. But under adverse conditions – famine, for example - more girls are born. While this girl/boy imbalance may not seem troublesome, think of the ramifications over a few generations. And, perhaps we need to connect the dots with the growing signs of dysfunction throughout our ecosystem?

As I see it, information is the key to waking up, to getting ourselves out of this biological experiment, as Dr. Salford and Professor Johansson have cautioned us.

Neurological Issues

Alzheimer's, dementia, Parkinson's Disease, ALS and MS may also be related to EMR, according to neuroscientists who explain this exposure can cause levels of neurotransmitters such as acetylcholine to drop abnormally. Low levels of acetylcholine are linked to a number of these neurological and neuromuscular symptoms and disorders.

(A side note: many people with these conditions improve dramatically when they deal with heavy metal toxicity and avoid artificial sweeteners such as those found in diet pop. Research the health effects of Aspartame, for example.)

You may not want to hear this; I know I didn't. While Alzheimer's Disease and dementia have generally been diseases of the elderly, based on the evidence of EMR biological harm, some experts are predicting these conditions will be afflicting people decades earlier.

The Silent Epidemic

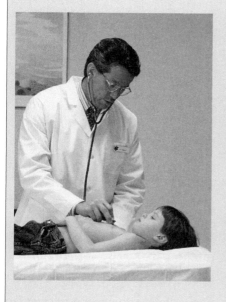

The young boy lies on the examining table banging his legs in an odd rhythm. He seems off in his own world. Standing close by, his parents look stunned: the pediatrician has just told them their child has autism.

They have known for a long time that something was not right but nothing prepared them for the raw shock of the diagnosis they had feared.

He had been such a healthy baby, and a normally developing toddler. Not long after his second birthday, however, they began to notice it was difficult to get him to focus, the development of his speech slowed, and he had occasional intense tantrums and hyperactivity.

They were taking extra steps to protect him, including having a new digital wireless baby monitor on at all times, close to where he sleeps. They kept his environment as clean and germ-free as they could with highly effective cleaning products.

Then they hear about a possible connection with the levels of microwave radiation from cell towers and wireless devices, including baby monitors. This possible link makes more sense when they read about an encouraging study: children like their son have done well in a low EMR environment. They decide to learn everything they can.

ADD/ADHD and Autism Spectrum Disorders

If you are facing these challenges you don't need anyone to tell you how difficult this can be, especially in the initial stages.

However, many families, through their courage and determination to find out as much as they can, are improving other parents' success in helping their children. Truly dedicated parents who are leading support and advocacy networks are helping a great many families.

This section includes the research and recommendations of several leading experts in this field.

Here's what I've discovered: what most people call autism is a wide and varied range of neurological conditions with symptoms that may include difficulty communicating and functioning socially, various developmental disabilities, and cognitive challenges. Some people on the Autism Spectrum also have extraordinary musical or mathematical skills.

Not long ago I met a remarkable young boy who introduced himself right away, announcing, "My name is David and I have OCD (obsessive-compulsive disorder) and Asperger's."

His eyes were bright and alert; he was obviously highly intelligent, and he seemed agitated. David then became distressed when someone asked me about the book I was writing on the health effects of electromagnetic radiation.

"Radiation?" he squealed, "Oh no. I don't want to know about that. That's too scary."

Many well-controlled adults have had the same reaction, but this vulnerable boy was visibly distraught. I shifted gears immediately and sat down with him and his mother, to listen to his fears, and do what I could to calm him. He appeared to feel better when we talked about all the ways we can be safer.

Evidently, David's parents had recently installed a DECT 6.0 cordless phone in his bedroom; he told me that he loves to talk for hours with his friends. He is a talented musician who spends many hours on an electronic keyboard, as well as a wireless laptop. Being environmentally concerned, the parents had switched all the lights in the house to compact fluorescents.

David's mother had just got the new high-powered 'smart' cell phone, with wireless headset, and told me that she had it on most of the day, and that it was often charged on standby in their bedroom at night – "just in case there's an important call".

She had been considering getting her son a cell phone as "it would be helpful to know where he was, and so he could call us if he was in trouble".

Having read this far in the book, are you also concerned about this child, and many like him?

It seems a great deal of research still needs to be done into the ways EMR exposure, and heavy metal toxicity, may affect normal neurological development in children like David.

What are some researchers and clinicians telling us now?

There seems to be no medical consensus on what causes autism and other seemingly brain-based disorders like ADHD, or how best to treat them. Many researchers say there are probably genetic factors that predispose a child to such conditions. But some are now piecing together a disturbing picture of how environmental toxins, heavy metals, molds, chemical/food sensitivities, infections, viruses, and EMR exposure can combine to create symptoms.

As you've seen in the symptoms chart a few pages back, concentration problems and hyperactivity are among the symptoms of electro-sensitivity, so it may well be that many thousands of children are being diagnosed and treated with drugs when removing them from EMR exposure could help them significantly.

Even children who don't have neurological problems can find it difficult to sit down, focus and succeed at school when there is a lot of EMR in the environment. (So why are so many schools installing wireless Internet?)

Some of the research that's coming in suggests a link: an American and Danish team of university researchers studied 13,000 young mothers who used cell phones during pregnancy. Their results, published in an epidemiology journal in 2008, found these women's children had a 50% higher than usual incidence of hyperactive behavior and emotional problems.

Having read this far, you are probably now aware that the radiation from the mothers' cell phones is likely only one factor.

A hospital in San Diego, California, found that 14 out of a group of 18 autistic children studied had lesions in the brain identical to those in rats exposed to low electro-magnetic frequencies between one and six days after birth.

The medical pioneer, Dietrich Klinghardt MD, PhD, is a physician who believes that the increase in autism is connected to the proliferation of EMR and our increasingly toxic environment.

In his ground-breaking work, Dr. Klinghardt is finding out how to recognize and treat the effects of toxic EMR on the genes of a developing fetus.

The hope is to prevent neurological and other problems from developing in the child.

In a recent interview, Dr. Klinghardt told me:

> In 10 of our autistic children we measured the EMR exposure of the mother in the location where she was sleeping before giving birth to the child – who later on would be diagnosed as autistic.
>
> We measured body voltage and microwave exposure from ambient background cell phone radiation.
>
> The results clearly showed significantly increased levels of EMF exposure in the affected mothers versus the control group.

Dr. Klinghardt has developed an approach to assessing exposure:

> We also take EMF/EMR measurements at the home (and whenever possible work location or school of children

with ADHD, behavioral problems, developmental delay and in adults with severe neurologic disease (Parkinson's, ALS, etc.) and the results are similar: the higher the exposure at home and at work, the more therapy-resistant or severe the illness.

The promising news is that many children are showing significant improvement in their symptoms, thanks to treatments that include: detoxification; supplementation with vitamins, antioxidants and cellular nutrients; dealing with food allergies and chemical sensitivities; infrared saunas, and a low EMF/EMR environment.

Katharina Gustavs adds, "As long as the infrared sauna being used is not a magnetic field hot spot."

Dr. Klinghardt's suggestions for reducing EMR exposure are not difficult and are affordable for most people. Here is the short list that is given to his patients, including those with ASD (autism):

a. no wireless technology and no cordless phones in the home (get wired broadband and corded phones)

b. switch off all fuses at night (unless you can measure body voltage and get specific)

c. use the sleep sanctuary principle: a silver coated mosquito net over the bed as a Faraday cage (greatly decreases microwave exposure)

Gustavs comments on using shielding fabric, "First, the electric fields in the room have to be measured – and reduced – to make sure they are not drawn into the Faraday cage increasing the radiation exposure."

Chris Anderson adds, "Please do the research and be cautious of what RF shielding fabric you purchase. There are cheaper varieties that tend to become brittle and shed off tiny particles of the metals used in the fabric, which can find their way into food and bodies and cause harm."

Generation Rescue, an international movement of scientists and physicians researching the causes and treatments for autism, ADHD and chronic illness, is aware of this issue:

> Our community is very concerned about the effects of Electromagnetic Radiation (EMR) on the body and how it deregulates the ability to manage toxins and infections, and how it seems to interfere with blood flow in the brain. We feel that Dr. Crofton's approach to reducing EMR exposure should be looked at by all families looking to raise a healthy child.

While evidence of the link between EMR and autism is still evolving, the experts I consulted praise the benefits of *all* children spending less electronic time, and more time discovering the simple wonders of nature.

Is your son or daughter mostly an 'inside', or 'outside', child?

Children With Autism Symptoms Benefit From A Low EMR Environment

This interesting and hopeful case study comes from Larry Gust, the electrical engineer and certified IBE environmental health consultant based in California:

> In mid 2008 I was called by a client with two children who were diagnosed with high heavy metals concentrations – particularly mercury. There was a 5 year-old boy with autism, and his sister, 3 years old, was behaviorally normal.
>
> Under medical supervision various strategies were tried to remove this toxic load from the children's bodies, but the results (monitored via urine analysis) were poor. A full environmental assessment of the house showed the principal issues were electromagnetic pollution from:

- A wireless Internet connection.

- A 5.8 GigaHertz cordless phone system.

- AC Magnetic field level of more than 3 milliGauss in the girl's bedroom.

- AC electric field of more than 7 Volts/metre in all bedrooms.

These changes were recommended:

- Eliminate the wireless Internet and cordless phone system and replace these with hard-wired Internet connections, and corded landline phones.

- Locate and repair wiring errors causing high magnetic field.

- At night, turn off the circuit breakers identified as causing the high electric field level in all the bedrooms.

> Just before these changes were implemented, the children had a urine test to determine if heavy metal were being eliminated from the body to the urine. There was little evidence of mercury dumping.

> One month after the changes another test was conducted. Mercury dumping doubled and uranium was showing up in the urine as well. By late fall 2008 the son was doing better than he had ever done in all aspects including behavior and his ability to learn.

Perhaps this is the picture: lower EMR = increase in heavy metal release = reduction in autism symptoms.

This is what's called anecdotal evidence, as you may know. Scientifically, this is not considered significant; it is, however, if it is your child who is getting better!

Connecting the dots again, this is interesting in light of the theory that EMR compresses the cell membrane affecting the transport channels, and inhibiting the release of toxins, including heavy metals.

EMR, Mercury and Autism?

You will notice that words like detoxification and mercury come up in this discussion on autism. This may come as a surprise to many researchers.

The still-forming picture of this mechanism is information that may benefit everyone who has issues with heavy metal toxicity, and may shed a new light on autism and other neurological disorders.

In his book, *From Fatigued to Fantastic,* Dr. Teitelbaum describes how the cell membrane works:

> All cells in the body are enclosed in a cell membrane, a balloon-like wall... Stiff cell walls can make it hard for cell membranes to perform their critical functions.

As I outlined earlier, researchers tell us when cells are exposed to EMR they go into a protective mode to ward off this foreign invader. Part of the reaction is compression of the cell membrane, making it rigid; this affects the in-flow of nutrients and out flow of toxins and waste products. This makes it difficult for cells to clear the mercury and other heavy metals.

Remember our river of health. With increased EMR exposure, the cells are not able to clear toxins properly, as we continue to dump more into the river, including repeated doses of mercury.

Boyd Haley, PhD, is the former chairman of the Department of Chemistry at the University of Kentucky and a National Institutes of Health post-doctoral scholar at Yale University Medical School.

Dr. Haley's research into the biochemical abnormalities found in people with Alzheimer's disease led to his identifying mercury toxicity as a major factor. He was one of the first to suggest that Thimerosal, the mercury-based preservative in infant vaccines, was possibly involved in autism-related disorders. This is highly controversial, as you may know.

A child can also be exposed to mercury prenatally, through the mother's mercury amalgam dental fillings, or later on if the child gets amalgam fillings. Heavy metal exposure can also come from the environment, as in the case of eating fish, particularly tuna, from contaminated waters.

According to Dr. Klinghardt and others who treat ASD, it appears that people with a genetic predisposition to autism have trouble clearing heavy metals from their cells.

An explanation for this, offered by some scientists, is that when a child's blood-brain barrier is more fully formed – around the age of 18 months – it can make it extremely difficult for the mercury from the vaccines received up until that date, and presumably any other heavy metal overload, to be excreted from the brain cells.

Dr. Jerry Kartzinel, MD, is a pediatrician who co-wrote, with Jenny McCarthy, the information-packed book, *Healing and Preventing Autism* (see Books in Resources, under Jenny McCarthy). Dr. Kartzinel explains why some children seem to be able to detox themselves from metal exposures – and not develop symptoms of autism – while others can't:

> We have natural pathways that are designed to clear toxic metals from our body. We are all born with different capacities to accomplish this. Some of our population is more easily poisoned than others. We know the very young and the very old are especially sensitive to poisonings and heavy metal…if they were never exposed to toxins

in the womb, they might never have had a problem. If they were exposed to just 'regular' toxins of day-to-day living, they would be fine.

Remember, we are speaking of a total body burden of heavy metals and toxins. This burden starts just after conception. By the time these babies take their first breath, their ability to mitigate the damage of toxic exposures is already taxed. Some children are barely taxed. Some children are almost maximally taxed. Those children born with a robust ability to detoxify sail right through. For others, though, clinical signs and symptoms start becoming evident at a very young age.

Even if your family is not dealing with any challenge of hyperactivity/autism, don't you find the increasing incidence disturbing? I do. Even if the human side of this epidemic does not unsettle you, just imagine the millions of dollars spent on assessment, treatment and support services.

Wouldn't it make sense to explore all avenues to seek the cause and cure of these conditions?

It seems to me that children with these neurological symptoms/conditions should be at the forefront of our efforts to reduce the EMR and other toxic exposures in our homes, schools, health care facilities and communities.

Detoxification

In *The Magnesium Miracle,* Dr. Carolyn Dean describes the many benefits of magnesium, including the process of detoxification and the ability of heavy metals to be released through the cell membrane:

> Magnesium is crucial for the removal of toxic substances and heavy metals such as aluminum and lead.

This is interesting in terms of the treatment of autism; I have also heard that magnesium is being used by some clinicians for EHS patients as it 'softens the cell membrane'.

Dr. Scheiner agrees detoxification is a key element in helping the body withstand even quite severe environmental assaults. He points out that while people in Finland were heavily exposed to radiation from the nuclear meltdown in Chernobyl, they had far lower levels of radiation sickness, and cancer, than you would expect. That's because, he says, the Finns' lifestyle includes saunas.

Sweating is one of the body's best mechanisms for clearing toxins. These specialists recommend the far infrared sauna – it seems more effective at detoxifying and you don't get as overheated as with a regular sauna. As you'll have figured out by now, you want to sit away from the electric element and find a lower EMR model. See the Resources Section.

Dr. Teitelbaum also offers a key to detoxification and/or buffering the effects of EMR with advice on the normal functioning of the cell membrane:

> This cell membrane is made up of fatty acids and a phosphorus molecule. Your body likes to use Omega-3

and -6 fatty acids when it makes cell membranes. When these are not available, your body has to use saturated fats and this results in rigid, poorly-functioning cellular walls. Essential fatty acids (EFAs) Omega-3 and -6 fatty acids play an important part here in keeping the cell membrane optimally functioning. This is particularly important when people are under severe physical stress or have increased sensitivities, including those sensitive to EMR. It is recommended to supplement even a healthy diet with good quality Omega-3 and -6 fatty acids."

While the comprehensive protocol combining the recommendations from all of our contributing experts is still a work in progress, there are many useful tips, including the benefits of magnesium from Dr. Dean, the essential fatty acids from Dr. Teitelbaum, the benefits of antioxidants from Dr. Scheiner and the therapeutic role of supervised detoxification from Dr. Klinghardt.

Nutritional Supplementation

Not all supplements are created equal, as you may know. Many are not absorbed by the cells of the body and quite literally go right through you. And with what we have learned about how EMR compresses the cell membrane, it is an even greater challenge for nutrients to be absorbed. I have heard some are working on supplements that can soften the cell membrane, including some forms of magnesium.

Dr. Scheiner also suggests several ways to strengthen and protect our immune system and overall health with supplements:

First, avoid exposure of environmental pollutants, as much as possible. This will help get rid of excess free radicals. To combat these we need scavengers

– antioxidant vitamins. It is not possible to get all the nutrients we need from even the healthiest diet. Our nourishment is losing antioxidants because of industrial agriculture. These days a strawberry has only 20% of its original amount of vitamin C. Therefore, it is necessary to use supplements including antioxidants, vitamins D and E, as well. All these water soluble vitamins don't enter the brain so we need scavengers that can pass the blood-brain barrier – melatonin, for example.

Other Key Health Factors

We've heard the experts talk about all the factors working together in a negative way, harming our health. But we can also combine many factors to contribute positively to our family's wellbeing, by boosting our bodies' abilities to buffer the electro-magnetic load we experience every day. After you have reduced your EMR, and some chemical, exposures, here are effective ways to boost your overall wellness and ability to deal with the EMR load on your system that you cannot control. Some physicians offer recommendations that can enhance your family action plan; they have become central to ours. We begin with dental health.

Dental Health

Dr. Klinghardt is only one of the physicians testing patients for heavy metal toxicity as one of the underlying causes of electro-sensitivity, Chronic Fatigue Syndrome, autism and many other conditions. Research the work of Dr. Boyd Haley, as well. This is the focus of many complementary medicine clinics, including that of Dr. Thomas Rau, the Swiss physician. Dr. Rau advises:

A strategy to consider for those experiencing electrical sensitivity symptoms is to remove the electromagnetic 'hot spot' in the head created by the presence of metal fillings.

Concern is thus not only for the neurotoxic aspect of mercury in fillings, an increasingly understood hazard, but because fillings themselves act as antennas in the presence of electromagnetic fields.

Dr. Rau says the removal of dental fillings can be an important early step in reducing electrical sensitivity, allowing some people to live in homes they otherwise could not tolerate.

(NOTE: removal of mercury fillings must be done by a dentist using a strict protocol, otherwise you, and the dentist, will be exposed to the mercury during the removal process. You must receive supplemental air during the procedure, I am told.)

Dr. Myron Wentz, a medical research scientist with a doctorate in microbiology and immunology, is also an internationally recognized virologist and cell biologist. Dr. Wentz is the founder of the comprehensive medical clinic, Sanoviv. Dr. Wentz has written a book detailing his concerns, *A Mouth Full of Poison*, (Medicis, S.C. 2004):

Today we know that mercury is the most toxic, non-radioactive heavy metal on the planet. Despite its toxicity, mercury is still used in manufacturing including the production of: batteries, thermometers, barometers, semi-conductors, electronic instruments, lighting and chemicals.

Mercury exposure, even at very low levels, diminishes the ability of the immune system to meet the slightest challenge. The number of T cells in the blood declines markedly when mercury amalgam is placed in the teeth, and the cells have now been programmed to undergo apoptosis – cellular death – in the presence of this mercury.

If you have personally decided to get vaccinated, or are required to do so, I urge you to opt for the nasal mist rather than the injectable vaccine. The nasal mist is free of mercury-containing thimerosal and is the natural route for administering a vaccine for a respiratory virus.

Biological Dentistry

John Snively, DDS, practised 25 years as a Biological Dentist incorporating complementary modalities of homeopathy, detoxification, supplementation and energetic medicine. Dr. Snively explains this approach:

> Toxic metals and other materials often become implanted in our teeth resulting in a long term burden to our immune system and root canals can also have devastating effects. The teeth and jaw joint provide us with a valuable sense of proprioception and discrepancies here can manifest throughout the body.

> Dissimilar metals in the mouth can create not only an electrical current but can also act as an antenna for other invisible Electromagnetic and Microwave forces.

In seeking a Biological Dentist one must first be certain that the office is "mercury free" and provides protection not only for you as a patient but that the dental team is wearing appropriate masks when removing toxic metals.

Some sort of biocompatibility testing should be offered to determine which materials are most tolerable for your immune system. Clifford Consulting & Research, of Colorado Springs, offers this testing – a dental materials screening. (www.ccrlab.com)

Safeguarding Your Family's Health the Holistic Way

As you may know, the complementary medicine approach has a lot to offer those of us who want to protect our families' health in this increasingly irradiated world. Complementary health practitioners tend to focus more on prevention and natural remedies such as those advocated by Dr. Andrew Weil and the others mentioned in this book, whereas the conventional medical model uses more pharmaceuticals to treat disease.

In this emerging field of electro-sensitivity it seems crucial to understand the complementary approach, as there are no drugs to treat this condition, and many conventional tests and treatments may exacerbate symptoms and conditions rather than improve them.

Dr. Scheiner describes the electro-sensitive person who's experiencing a range of symptoms when exposed to these frequencies. Unfortunately, this percentage of the population is growing dramatically in virtually every corner of the world. Few people, and few of their doctors, recognize these symptoms and their potential cause.

Therefore, after many medical or non-medical tests and therapies, patients' symptoms may remain and over the long term even worsen, as they have not been able to identify and treat the source. For some, the source is the invisible waves of radiation that surrounds us all.

The best possibility here is that people have recognized their body's wireless wake-up call, are hearing the body's alarm, and taking steps to avoid the exposure.

While many people are suffering, with their daily activities severely limited, feeling overwhelmed and victimized by the electro-pollution, in some ways these canaries in the coal mine may be doing better than the miners, who are also being exposed and affected, but do not hear

and/or heed the symptoms.

One of the main objectives of this book, and my new health advocacy, is to get the word out that if you're having a lot of trouble sleeping, if you're fatigued, having skin tingling, burning sensations, difficulty focusing, any light-headedness or dizziness, this collection of symptoms may well be your body's attempt to let you know that this exposure is harmful.

Dr. Scheiner's observation:

> Each symptom, like the headaches, sleep disruption, dizziness etc. can be unspecific – caused by a lot of different reasons. It gets specific, however, when you experience several of these – this could be what we're calling microwave syndrome – this is not a sickness, it is a warning system.
>
> Your body is trying to alert you, saying, 'I'm having trouble here, get me out of this situation'. These symptoms are a call for help. As you may know, in our conventional medical system, it is often our approach to deal with these symptoms, in a sense trying to shut the body up, masking the calls for help and giving relief of the symptoms.
>
> The cause of the distress, however, may not be addressed and therefore continues the harm. What we see, clinically, is that this can progress to more serious conditions.

I've had the good fortune to have several transatlantic conversations with Dr. Hans Scheiner, and the more I hear from him of how EMR affects the cells and stresses the body, the more it reminds me of much of the work I had been doing in emotional and physical stress.

In my previous book, *The Healthy Type A*, I developed an Early Stress Warning cue to help people tune into this stress reaction sooner, giving themselves greater success at reducing this potentially harmful response.

With Dr. Scheiner's inspiration, I began to develop an exercise to recognize the early symptoms of EMR exposure.

Radiation Rescue Early Warning Cue

This is an exercise where you take note of the first signs – the slight tingling, the slight light-headedness, etc. It is much easier to deal with these symptoms when they are just beginning, as you would assume.

This early indicator can serve as a cue, an alert to wake you up that you need to do something about where you are right now.

When you recognize this cue, the first obvious step is to reduce the exposure. For example, are you in a wireless hot spot? Has your neighbor installed a new router; have you up-graded the cordless phone model?

You might go back to the questionnaire in Strategy 2 and look at the symptoms you checked off. Then note the ones that seem to occur first. These can become your early warning cues.

When you recognize this cue, you know it is time to get away from what you are doing, and where you are, if you can. This is where an EMR detector is so helpful. It can alert you to high EMR areas, and also to lower ones you can seek when you recognize your cue.

Getting outside, away from electronics, is often good, unless you are close to power lines, masts or cell tower antennas.

Having a cool, or warm, shower can be helpful. And being beside a waterfall, fountain, stream, river, or ocean can be restorative.

Now let's take a look at a variety of ways we can protect and restore our health – our greatest treasure, as you know.

Health and Wellbeing Strategies

Grounding Exercises

A physician who specializes in energy medicine told me that he advises his electro-sensitive patients to remember the healing, restorative power of nature. This is not as far-out as you might imagine. Remember what Dr. Becker told us about the natural electro-magnetic fields of the earth.

This doctor recommends going outside and standing barefoot on the actual earth, if at all possible (sand, dirt, grass are best, but if pavement is all you've got, it'll do).

Lean or crouch over so that all your fingers touch the ground. If you're feeling light-headed or dizzy, you might need support. He suggests doing some relaxed deep-breathing, and feel as much as you can that you are reconnecting with the earth and the natural energies around you. The surgeon Dr. Rea also recommends this grounding practice.

There are explanations for this grounding – it might be that with hands and feet both on the ground you're completing a circuit and allowing the buildup of artificial electro-magnetic energy in your body to be discharged into the earth.

Dr. Sinatra has written *Earthing* (Basic Health Publications, 2010 with Clinton Ober and Martin Zucker) on the physiological benefits of grounding. As you may know, what Dr. Sinatra calls "good vibes" can heal and balance us when we connect with the harmonious forces of the natural world – walking barefoot on the earth is the best way.

Dr. Sinatra explains:

> Our research has shown that these grounding exercises can calm and balance our systems and produce a physiological shift from the sympathetic nervous system (stress mode) to the parasympathetic (relaxation mode). The results of this shift have a positive effect on many cardiovascular risk factors: thickened blood was normalized, heart function was balanced, there was a reduction in oxidative stress from free radicals easing the disruption of blood vessels, inflammation was reduced, and there was an easing of anxiety. These are significant health benefits.

Another good way to ground: pause and take a few deep breaths, letting go as you exhale. Not heavy breathing and hyperventilating; it's more changing the way you breathe – lower and deeper with the abdomen moving. With each inhalation, focus on breathing in energizing oxygen, and with each exhalation, expelling stale air, and some of your stress. More on this coming up in a few pages.

Anti-aging – Important New Discoveries

No other generation has faced our health challenges; we need to adapt. This is one focus of Dr. Sinatra, who is a founding member of the American Academy of Anti-Aging Medicine (A4M). Both of us speak at the annual conference. As we've said, EMR has been shown to: impair DNA repair and other cellular and organ functions; decrease memory; suppress immunity; diminish melatonin and cause sleep problems; affect eyesight, and increase inflammation – primary aging factors. As Dr. Blank's research shows, living amidst the increasing smog of electro-pollution also produces unhealthy stress on our cells.

And remember the German study that found EMR exposure impaired our neurotransmitters – the electric impulses in the brain. Not good! So each step you take in this plan brings a wealth of anti-aging benefits.

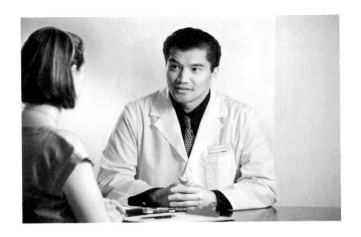

I hope this book inspires you to take better care of your body's electrical system – your heart and nervous system. This is critical as we age. I highly recommend tai chi and chi gong. These practices have been used for thousands of years to balance and ground our life force energy, and promote longevity and lifelong wellness. These ancient spiritual and health belief systems completely understood "the body electric" – hence the development of acupuncture and other forms of energy medicine.

Acupuncture

Traditional Chinese Medicine (TCM) has its roots in Taoism. Its practitioners have known for at least five thousand years that the life energy of humans and other living creatures is connected with, and influenced by, the energies in our environment, whether these are natural or artificial. TCM practitioners see the human body in terms of a system of pathways, or meridians, through which our life force energy (called qi, or chi) travels. Our health depends on the balanced and unhindered flow of this energy.

Dr. Hong Zhen Zhu, author of *Building a Jade Screen: Better Health with Chinese Medicine* (Penguin Canada 2001), has treated a number of patients with EMR-related symptoms. Although EMR is a relatively new kind of assault on our bodies' natural electro-magnetic energies, Dr. Zhu applies classical TCM theory to what he's observed in his patients' symptoms.

Dr. Zhu explains:

> EMR disrupts the normal direction of energy flow along the meridians, affecting many body systems and functions. It also disturbs mental functioning, mood and spirit. Acupuncture is helpful in treating the brain fog, insomnia, and other EMR-related conditions such as Chronic Fatigue Syndrome and sensitivity to noise and light.

Dr. Zhu also recommends such mind-body balancing practices as tai chi, chi gong and meditation.

Dr. Carrie Hyman, LAc, OMD, a licensed acupuncturist and Doctor of Chinese Medicine, recommends specific herbs and antioxidants:

> A TCM practitioner can recommend Chinese Tonic herbs. These are a unique class of herbs that are preventative and restorative. The numerous benefits include adaptogenic properties. Many of these longevity enhancing "superior herbs", have been valued by the Chinese for thousands of years. Modern science reveals that they are high in polyphenols (green tea), flavonoids (berries...anti-inflammatory), polysaccharides and antioxidants. Moreover, they support the body's ability to manufacture endogenous antioxidants like SOD and glutathione peroxidase. This is important as EMFs increase free-radical – oxidative stress, thereby increasing our need for antioxidants.

NeuroModulation Technique, NMT

This is another treatment that works on the principles of energy medicine. NeuroModulation Technique (NMT) was developed by a chiropractor/complementary health practitioner, Dr. Leslie S. Feinberg, DC, in 2002. His website www.nmt.md describes this approach:

> The informational basis of illness and disease may be the most common, yet the most overlooked, roadblock to healing. NMT is best described as 'informational medicine,' because it works to identify and correct the informational source of illness – the confusion that can interrupt our innate healing mechanisms.

> Many people believe that illness results from some external affliction that viciously attacks the mind-body. The NMT position is that illness is the inevitable result of informational confusion and faults in the systems responsible for regulating body functions, making them unable to produce the balanced internal-body state that wellness requires.

> A good example of this is food allergy, where the immune system is so confused that the body damages itself by its misguided reaction to a food that it should see as beneficial nutrition. Seen in this light, illness or "disease" in the body happens by default when the mind-body is not sufficiently aware of its internal conditions and the requirements for healing.

> The mind-body is a self-correcting system that always seeks to find and maintain the balanced internal state in which optimal health and vitality thrive.

I asked Dr. Feinberg how this system might benefit people with EMR exposure symptoms and conditions:

> With thermal exposure there is obvious harm – heating of the tissue. As you have told me, most of the concern in the scientific community is with non-thermal levels from cordless and cell phones, Wi-Fi etc., where the radiation is not strong enough to heat tissue, but is causing harm nonetheless. We could use the analogy of allergy and toxicity. Mercury is highly toxic – harmful to everyone. This could be compared to thermal EMR exposure. An allergy, however, happens when the immune system is provoked to react in an 'inappropriate' way, causing reaction symptoms – inflammation etc. This could be compared to what happens on the cellular level with non-thermal EMR exposure. Perhaps it is not so much that this level of radiation is harmful to the body, as it is confusing.

Confusing? I remembered what I had heard about the mechanism of harm – the cell membrane going into 'lockdown' mode as it does not recognize these new artificial frequencies – and that it was this reaction (misinterpretation) that affected the normal functioning of the cell.

I found this conversation with Dr. Feinberg illuminating and encouraging. You can imagine what it has been like for me to be immersed in this issue for the past four years, reading more and more research that presents increasingly troubling results. I asked Dr. Feinberg how this 'confusion' might explain electro-sensitive people. He said that some people are very reactive and have symptoms. With electro-sensitive people it might be tingling of the skin, headaches, difficulty sleeping etc.

Remember what Dr. Scheiner told us about people becoming "allergic" to electricity?

But what about something like leakage of the blood-brain barrier? I asked Dr. Feinberg. Although this specific area has not been the main focus of Dr. Feinberg's work, and he was not familiar with Dr. Salford's research, he replied that this could be explained by inflammation – one of the body's primary reactions.

I wanted to three-way Professor Salford into the conversation right away, and to bring in all our other experts. Hopefully, one day we can get these researchers and clinicians together to provide a more complete picture of how this all works, and how best to diagnose and treat EMR exposure. Not only for the millions of electro-sensitive people, but for all those with high EMR exposure who have not yet developed symptoms.

NMT and Autism

Dr. Feinberg told me that NMT was used recently in a research study with children with autism, led by Dr. Robert Weiner, a Clinical Psychologist in Dallas, Texas. The trial was stopped after 18 children completed the study.

The results were so positive that Dr. Weiner wanted to report the findings as soon as possible rather than waiting another 6-12 months to collect more data before he announced the findings and published the study. Dr. Weiner designed the study to determine the effectiveness of NMT in improving the functioning of children with autism. The study ran for 12 sessions over 6 weeks. Statistically significant improvement was noted by the end of 6 sessions, with continued improvement occurring through the end of the study.

Parents whose children were in the study were amazed at the changes they saw in their children during the course of the study. Each session averaged 45 minutes, so the study demonstrated that NMT was able to produce profound changes in these children in a total of only 9 hours of NMT treatment.

This is a small study, with encouraging results. We need to help these families get their children back so they can all thrive.

I wanted to call Dr. Klinghardt right away to tell him this news. Then Dr. Feinberg told me that Dr. Klinghardt knows his work, so is probably already aware of this study and its promising results.

I was "connecting the dots" during this conversation and saw a comparison, not only with allergies, but with the "miscommunication" of the fight or flight response – the source of our emotional stress. This is when the body gets all geared up – muscles tighten, blood pressure goes up, etc. – with our basic instincts to fight that tiger, when the only threat is slow traffic.

Another Key Factor – Your Acid-Alkaline (pH) Balance

There is a Swiss naturopathic doctor who specializes in this area. Dr. Christopher Vasey ND, in his book, *The Acid-Alkaline Diet*, explains why this balance is so important to overall health, and why most of us are overly acidic. Not good news: most of the foods in our

Western diet are highly acidic – meats, starchy foods (white-floured pasta), sugars (most fruits, all cakes, cookies, sodas etc.) alcohol and, of course, vinegar. Dr. Vasey reports that fatigue is a primary symptom of being overly acidic.

Other symptoms include: irritability, depression, headaches, inflamed gums, skin inflammation, red blotches, itching, heartburn and other stomach and digestive problems, excessive urination, fungal diseases (yeasts thrive in the acidic environment), joint and muscle pain and our old friend insomnia.

This list reminds me of the Chronic Fatigue and the EMR checklists. It may seem puzzling; however, everything is interconnected in our body. And when the natural balance of this vital pH is thrown off, it affects all the fluids and systems in the body, producing many symptoms.

Briefly: Dr. Vasey describes effective ways to test urine and saliva – good indicators – and how to bring the pH back into healthy balance. All green and colored vegetables – without any sweet or sour sauces – are the primary alkalizing foods and should be included in every main meal, he recommends. This doesn't mean we give up acidic foods like meat, sugar and many grains; it does mean that we balance with alkalizing foods: vegetables, green drinks, soft cheeses, almonds and avocados.

Keeping Hydrated

This is vital. Virtually every complementary medicine practitioner highly recommends that we drink lots of pure water. Sorry, this does not include coffee, tea, juice, soda or alcohol. This means good, filtered H_2O. Every cell and system in the body must have sufficient toxin-free water to maintain healthy functions.

And this is crucial for any kind of detoxification. It is also helpful in terms of our EMR exposure, as much of our cells' composition, and our cell membranes, are lipids and liquid and need to stay permeable, as Dr. Teitelbaum explained.

Here's a good tip: drink your large glass of water, with alkalizing greens, between meals. There are also mineral drops and powders that you can add to alkalize your system. It is best to hydrate and alkalize *between* meals, not with them, as you don't want to dilute your digestive enzymes. It is also good *not* to drink ice water with meals, as this hampers digestion.

Techno Speed, Stress and Everyday Frenzy

Are you discovering there are many facets to this discussion, not just health concerns? All these electro-seductions can grab our attention by the throat and not let go. I read that when we are staring at a computer screen, we blink a fraction of the times we should. Ever felt dizzy at the keyboard when you realize you have been so ramrod focused that you forgot to breathe?

We may tell ourselves, "take breaks, breathe, stretch", yet the hours go by and we're hunched up, tightened up and bleary-eyed, still staring at the screen. It's as though we've lost touch with the fact that we have a body, until we notice the aching low back, sore neck and shoulders and wrist pain. Some people even think computering can be good down time. The hyper-speed that all this technology affords us is a two-edged convenience. People used to have to wait for you to return messages; now, they demand instant access.

And there used to be quiet moments in our day – waiting for the kids after school, waiting for a bus, or just hanging out. Now, we never have to be alone. There never has to be a gap. We can fill every bit of space with texting, if we can't be talking or shopping online. This can lead to a very speedy mind. Our dazzling display of technology feeds right into, we could almost say enables, unhealthy stress.

Remember Toad of Toad Hall, in *The Wind In The Willows?* How he would have loved instant messaging and video gaming. Zooming from one call to the next can feel so exhilarating. We hardly need to take a breath in between.

All this speed can make us feel so alive; it is, however, hard on the system. When the body responds with a surge of adrenaline, heart rate and rhythm are disrupted, blood pressure goes up, the blood thickens – not a good combination – muscles tighten, the normal functioning of immune and gastro-intestinal systems is suppressed, and more.

Foolishly, the body thinks these responses are going to save us from that saber-toothed tiger, when in fact, these 'adaptations' work against us. (Reminds me of the theory of the cell membrane's misunderstanding of non-thermal EMR exposure.)

This misplaced stress response disturbs our sleep, makes us tense, ages us more rapidly and can lead to a wide range of symptoms and conditions. You know this feeling – you're restless, edgy and impatient. It's not only the jet-fuel java accelerating your heart, it is also the stress response.

Our high-tech toys feed our Type A need for speed. I know this from my research, and personal experience: high-energy go-getters can be a tad impatient. I realize that this personality style plays a role here.

If we are going to reduce our EMR exposure, unhook ourselves from our tech obsession, it seems we need to cut this cycle of urgency, speed and stress. A challenge: do you know anyone who is not stressed these days?

Even vacations don't seem to provide much of a gap. Here's a good space-filler I saw recently: a luxury resort is now offering your own wireless television set, complete with wireless headsets, poolside. (No, I don't remember the name of it.) We can quite literally, go into withdrawal when someone, some thing attempts to take away our 'drug'. Try taking your child off computer games 'cold turkey', or forgoing texting, emailing, YouTubing, Facebooking and web-surfing for a day. We may need to come off slowly.

Whatever you can do to reduce the adrenaline will help. In fact, cutting back on caffeine – gradually, to avoid a withdrawal headache – is a very helpful way to slow you down and will make it easier to cut back on your tech time, assuming this is what you want to do.

Before you got caught up in this swirl, do you remember what more slow-paced pastimes you enjoyed? Reading? Walking in the park? Sitting on a log at the beach? Without headphones. Maybe visit a friend. Yes, actually, go and *see* them. And sit and chat. Reconnect. When we allow our mind to slow down, our body will follow. This is a good approach for digital detox.

There are some ways that we can enjoy these together. Meditation, for example. Just plain sitting. Being with your breath. Being with your mind. Being where you are. Unplugged. An outrageous thought, perhaps? To sit quietly. To tune in. To just take some down time to be with ourselves, to be with this moment, somehow goes against the grain in our modern world.

Calming the Scattered Mind

Interestingly, in Japan, one of the most frenetic cultures on this planet, many people still seek out the quiet contemplative environment of Zen meditation. Nothing religious, just taking time to slow down, and tune in.

I have studied meditation, flower arranging and Tea Ceremony for many years – an accomplishment for a go-getter. When I had a clinical practice and taught people progressive relaxation, I used to combine this with simple breath meditation. This was before we were so crazed and dazed by technology, so it is even more useful now to pull ourselves away from the screen, power off, and sit quietly for a few moments.

Dr. Jon Kabat-Zinn is the author of *Wherever You Go, There You Are: Mindfulness Meditation In Everyday Life* and founder of the Stress Reduction Clinic at the University of Massachusetts Medical Centre.

Dr. Kabat-Zinn describes what it is like to have a meditation practice:

> ... by making some time for this each day doesn't mean that you won't be able to think any more, or that you can't run around, or get things done. It means that you are more likely to know what you are doing because you have stopped for awhile and watched, listened, understood.

You can try this mindfulness meditation at any time of day.

Posture: Sit comfortably on a straight-backed chair or on a cushion on the floor. Let your shoulders relax and let your arms hang straight down by your sides. Rest your hands, palms down, comfortably on your legs.

Eyes: Your eyes are open – helpful in keeping from dozing off. Your gaze is soft and relaxed; you look out and down slightly.

Breath: try to refrain from fancy breathing. You are not trying to bliss out, or get caught up in any other entertainment. Just sit quietly and breathe normally. Once you settle a bit your breathing will become more natural. Just breathe in through your nose, and out through your nose. Let your jaw relax.

Attention: The challenge here is that the more you need to do this, the more difficult it may be. Some of us haven't sat quietly with ourselves for a long time. It's hard to grasp but the action here is to just be. Just let your attention rest on your breathing.

YOU ARE NOT TRYING TO STOP YOUR THOUGHTS!

This only creates more. Let the thoughts – and all those colorful emotions – come and go. When you wake up and realize that you have been carried away by them; come back. Come back to the gentle movement of the breath. This helps to train, focus and calm the mind.

The Benefit: What has this got to do with our Radiation Rescue? When we are no longer uneasy in the space of things as they are; no longer edgy when alone, or frantic when nothing is 'happening', we find ourselves spending more time away from the computer and our other diversions. And every moment we are unplugged reduces our EMR exposure.

When we get outside, just being in nature, our energy soars. And when we walk barefoot on the earth (or wearing unlined leather moccasins without rubber soles) we are grounding and enjoying many benefits. May I suggest you try this and see.

Yoga, Tai Chi and Other Body/Mind Practices

The benefits with these practices are numerous, in this context they help us reconnect with ourselves, ease the stress in our bodies, clear the clutter from our minds and release the stale breath from our lungs, as well as focus the mind. I'm sure you can find a good class at your local recreation center, if you want to try out these body/mind exercises.

These flowing activities, particularly when done out in the fresh air, and when we breathe deeply, helps to recharge our life force energy and helps us to reconnect with the natural energy fields of the earth.

Walk, Stretch, Swim, Enjoy

Remember the River of Health, and how it can be flowing or stagnant? An easy way to diagnose your own inner river is: if you feel tired and low energy, the flow is sluggish, toxins are building up, and you're lacking oxygen.

One of the best ways to recharge our EMR-overloaded systems is to get this river moving again; our blood moving, lymph flowing and chi circulating. Stretching at the keyboard is good for crunched muscles, but it's even better to get away from it.

You may have built up resistance; exercise being a way to lose weight. You may have come to resent feeling pressured into being fit. But let's look at being more active from a different perspective, one that is pivotal to staying healthy amidst environmental pollutants.

You don't have to walk, cycle or run for miles; just get a stagnant system moving. Flowing. The vitality of our lymph system is a key element in dealing with almost all of the symptoms and conditions we've been discussing.

If this clearing house is not functioning well there is a build-up of toxins, the immune system becomes overwhelmed and we are more likely to be sensitive to chemical and electro-pollution, have allergies and food sensitivities, among other problems. Being more physically active helps the lymphatic fluid clear toxins and this improves so many conditions.

A spry 90 year-old woman at our rec center coached me on her swim routine: warm up your muscles in the hot tub, take a brief cool shower, then swim. She does ten slow and steady laps, while I splash around in the aqua-fit class. After you get out of the pool, she suggests, have a steam to help the body flush out any toxins from the pool water. Some gentle stretching and re-hydrating with lots of pure water completes her routine. Try it.

When you recognize the Early Warning Cue which tells you that your stress, or EMR exposure, levels are rising, get up and get outside. Lie on the grass. Look off into the distance.

Watch birds in the sky.

This is good for eyes that spend long hours staring at various electronic screens. Swing your arms. Breathe deeply. Move.

This, and staying hydrated, are the best ways to keep the river flowing. Swim. Play tag with your children at the park. Put on your era's favorite music and dance just like you used to do. That will make them smile. I encourage you to add to your action plan twenty minutes daily of being outside in the fresh air. Feel too tired? All the more reason to get moving. You may find it more effective, and more fun, than the usual ways we try to deal with fatigue – the sugary carb, or the caffeine kick. (Isn't it annoying that many of the things that taste good aren't good for us?)

The Communication Challenge

Recognize this eye roll? Persuading supposedly rational adults to adopt a safer-tech lifestyle is one thing. How do you get your teens to understand that their beloved cell phone, so central to their social life, is as much of a safety issue as sex, drug use, wearing a helmet, driving safely and so on?

I spoke with Dr. Allison Rees, a counsellor and parenting expert, who agrees that dealing with this hyper-tech generation can be a real challenge:

Teens need and want to make their own decisions, just at a time when they aren't good at doing that! So we attempt to educate, state our concerns and negotiate, as best we can. I suggest not indulging children with the technology, and not seeing these devices as a privilege. I'm concerned with the sense of entitlement kids have around getting this 'stuff'.

Dr. Rees offers some ideas for communicating more effectively with your children, which may be helpful whether you're talking about technology, or any other issues.

Here are some of her key points:

- Say what you want to say; don't just react to the child's statements or behavior;

- Stay on one topic, be brief and to the point, and don't bring up issues from the past;

- Do respect the teen's need for independence and request a positive change;

- Don't lecture or try to control by making demands, commands, threats, or guilt-inducing statements, or fear-inducing warnings.

Dr. Rees adds:

> People, including children, tend to resist being pushed, coerced, or otherwise forced into changing their behavior. When a parent forces a child to change his or her behavior, the child reacts like someone whose head is held under water by a bigger, more powerful person. He/she does anything possible to resist. If the parent succeeds, the child feels resentful and wants revenge.

It is therefore important for us as parents to make requests rather than give orders. We should recognize that it's up to our children to control and change their behavior, rather than trying to impose such changes on them. Only in situations where there is actual physical danger should we try to control our children.

I would suggest that in the case of radiation exposure, as with other health and safety issues such as alcohol consumption and driving, you engage your teens in a problem-solving discussion around solutions that will keep them safer while still respecting their need for autonomy and some privacy. For instance, can they agree to abide by some of the safer use guidelines for cell phones – limiting use, keeping them powered off and away from their heads at night, and using the speakerphone or wired headset? As with so many issues that come up as our children grow into young adults, we have to be clear about our reasons and give them the information they need. As Dr. Rees reminds us, lecturing breeds resistance.

Other Technology Issues:

A Good Morning America segment interviewed five top texting teens – one boy sent up to 35,000 messages a month. I was amazed that his parents did not seem horrified with this saying, "Well, it doesn't seem to be affecting his school work".

Let's consider the radiation exposure. However, there are also concerns with teens and technology that go beyond physical health effects and distractions at school. For instance, vicious attacks of cyber-bullying, where a young teen is targeted with abusive emails or instant messages.

Or the obsession with texting which has developed a sideline where young people send each other nude photos of themselves by cell phone. Check in with your children and teens about their communications. Check the bill to see how often the phone is being used.

Internet Safety

If our children were confronted on the street, or in a video arcade, by the stranger they may be freely opening up to online, they might be horrified. And, perhaps, in danger. The health hazards of wireless radiation are not our only concern with all those hours spent online. No, it's not all homework. Ever notice that they suddenly switch screens when you walk in?

Last night we heard an Internet safety expert talk at our children's school – an eye opener for the parents and students. I asked Jesse Miller, founder and lead at Miller Consulting Services, for his insights:

> I am concerned about users who participate without regard for privacy and the personal repercussions of having an open profile. Everything you post: messages, pictures, videos etc. become the property of that website. And social networking websites are actively providing your personal information to other companies, with your approval based on agreement of the prescribed terms of use.

> Not knowing, and/or not caring, about any consequences, our youth see Facebook, for example, as a place where they can be who they are, communicate with friends openly, without adult judgement and make certain to stay in the loop about personal and world events.

> The consequences, however, to this behaviour when un-

monitored, or addressed by parents, can be detrimental to their endeavours in the future. Most young people, and adults, do not know that permanent traces are left behind. It is common for potential employers, school and university admissions to use Facebook, and other sites, in their screening process. The young people, and adults, I talk with assure me that their profile is closed and secure. This is not always the case. I show them how easy it is to access and retain their personal information, pictures etc.

Less common, but potentially serious and tragic, police investigations track home invasions, abductions, sexual assaults and homicides that have resulted from seemingly innocent online encounters. I encourage parents to explain to their children that their passwords should be available (maybe in a sealed envelope) as access to these accounts will be one of the first steps in a police investigation.

I advise parents to discuss online activities openly with their children and realize that what youth communicate in this way is no better and no worse than what previous generations did when their parents weren't looking, or listening. The difference is that today this personal information – including pictures, schools, home addresses, when you are home alone, away on holiday, and telephone numbers – is digitized through social networking multimedia and in turn being brought into public view, to anyone seeking it.

The Internet has many benefits. We do, however, need to use this resource more safely, and securely. (More details at www.howsafe.ca)

A computer expert from the Silicon Valley told me, "I don't do social networking. I know what they do with the data."

The Safer-Tech Family Challenge

Roberto Salti and colleagues at the University of Florence in Italy found that when 74 children, aged 6 to 12, were deprived of their TVs and computers for a week, and other sources of artificial light were reduced in their homes, there was a beneficial outcome: the production of melatonin increased by an average of 30 per cent. The increases were highest in the youngest children.

And as you may know, being outside in the sunshine triggers the internal production of Vitamin D, which is also essential to our health.

Ever wondered what might happen if your family were to unplug from the virtual world and reconnect? This is for families wired on wireless who want to reconnect with each other, and the natural world around us. If you've had children in primary schools, you might have participated in "turn off the TV week", when families are encouraged to spend time reading, playing games, listening to music, going outside – any activity that doesn't require a television or computer monitor.

There was a TV challenge some time ago for families to go without for a month. I remember one young teen complaining it "was like a death in the family". Interestingly, there were similar stages – irritation, boredom, anger and eventually, if they could hang in there, some times of once-lost fun and jokes. Some parents reported that it was really refreshing not to have to drag the kids away from the TV show or the "next level" in the video game when it's time for dinner.

I'd like to propose a similar experiment: a trial run at a safer-tech family life. Remember the joy of reading, books, the printed page?

Don't panic – you don't have to toss out all things electronic. I'm hoping this process will give you the time and mental space to see how much of the technology is really necessary in helping you function and stay connected, and how much is just a habit and mental clutter.

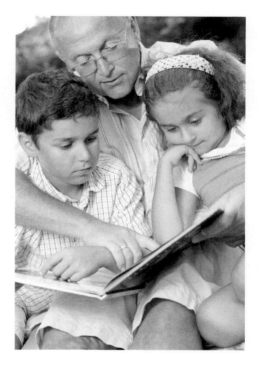

Take another look at the questionnaire to see how central technology is to your family's activities. In the evening is everyone in their own space texting, emailing, watching TV, playing video games? Isn't every family, you might ask?

There are many families, ours is one, who enjoy some "no-screen" evenings listening to music and reading, or playing cards, board games. Sharing laughs. Last Spring Break we went to a family resort that offers lots of outdoor activities. We were surprised that the nature trails were empty, while the parking lot was full. We had a wonderful time exploring the woodsy wonders below the forest's canopy, digging in the inter-tidal zone, splashing at the water's edge and sitting on logs watching birds. Does your family enjoy such wandering?

We have given our children hand-me-down digital cameras; this is a great way for them to develop an appreciation of nature, and have fun taking pictures and sharing them with friends. (Yes, most of the time on Facebook.) Reconnecting with each other doesn't have to be rare family holiday time, it could be part of your weekly life.

One Family's Safer-Tech Challenge:

Here's a follow-up with our 'library mum':

1. Thought about nature deprivation. We don't live near any woods but I unplugged the kids and went to the park the other day. Played and had a wonderful time.

2. Today, took the kids to the ocean...bypassed children's playground and went straight to tide pools and rocky shore. Had a great time with them exploring barnacles, shells and watching the tide...thought about nature deprivation and how wonderful it felt to be with them in this unscripted environment.

3. Thinking about how to redesign life in ways that aren't just about restricting or taking away toys/conveniences, but finding creative ways to do things that contribute to overall wellbeing...this is in response to my son who is concerned that our discussions will lead to the restriction of things that he loves (and it probably will, but he may end up happier as we spend more time outdoors in nature!)

It could make a powerful difference if more women were as quick to re-think their families' balance between nature and technology, as our library mum and her neighbour have. There was a recent article from

BBC news in the UK, reporting on a surging number of "geek mums". It seems many women are using their emails, cell phones, texting, Twittering, blogging, to counter the loneliness and social isolation of being at home with children.

Consider the fact that more than 60% of electronic devices are evidently purchased by women; you see the potential impact mothers, grandmothers, sisters, aunts can have on this issue, if they choose. It's quite amazing that a small shift in the family focus can bring great benefits. We haven't made any major changes – just less time on the computer – all of us that is, as I was spending a lot of time there myself writing this book. We are making an effort to get outside more, even in less than brilliant weather.

Our Children's Connection With Nature?

Have you heard that the latest version of the Oxford Junior Dictionary (Oxford University Press) has deleted nature words like: beaver, dandelion, heron, magpie, otter, acorn, clover, ivy, sycamore, willow and blackberry? In their place, they have substituted more popular terms, like the electronic "Blackberry", "blog", "MP3 player", and "broadband".

Canadian wildlife artist and conservationist Robert Bateman, whose "Get to Know Program" has been inspiring children to go outdoors and "get to know" their wildlife neighbors for more than a decade said in an interview with The Canadian Press:

If you can't name things, how can you love them? And if you don't love them, then you're not going to care a hoot about protecting them or voting for issues that would protect them.

If you are feeling inspired about changing direction with the focus of your family so they will have a greater appreciation of nature, and unplug now and then, I encourage you to approach this with tact.

As you know, it is not easy to guide your children in the direction you want them to grow. And it can be irritating, even heartbreaking, that they seem to insist on moving in the opposite direction – you want them to be playing outside in the fresh air, and they prefer being inside, glued to video games in darkened rooms.

Richard Louv, author of *Last Child In The Woods*, has a great quote in his book from a child who declared, with one of those looks, "Of course, I prefer to play inside. That's where all the electrical outlets are." This is funny, in a way. And tragic, in another. Richard shares his insights on saving our children from what he calls nature-deficit disorder:

> People around my age enjoyed a kind of free, natural play that seems, in the era of kid pagers, instant messaging, and Nintendo, like a quaint artifact.

> Within the space of a few decades, the way children understand and experience nature has changed radically. Today, kids are aware of the global threats to the environment – but their physical contact, their intimacy

with nature, is fading. Yet, at the very moment that the bond is breaking between the young and the natural world, a growing body of research links our mental, physical and spiritual health directly to our association with nature – in positive ways... The health of our earth is at stake.

Richard Louv goes on to inspire us about the possibility of a "new frontier – a better way to live with nature." His work has evolved into the much-heralded Children & Nature Network (www.childrenandnature. org) and the Leave No Child Inside program.

It's tempting to keep including quotes here from his wonderfully thought-provoking *Last Child in the Woods* (Algonquin Books, 2008.) This book offers so much great information that it is pivotal to our Safer-Tech Family Challenge.

What does your family love about being outside?

Here's a story of a neighbor, an overwhelmed dad – who is inspired to make some changes in his family's life.

When He Was a Boy

This dad became so electro-sensitive that he sought not only to regain his own health, but to prevent such a situation with his young family:

> When I was younger we were outside most of the time, except for those long hours in school. My friends and I used to make up games where we would roar around and using our imaginations in all sorts of scenarios. We discovered how things worked by putting things together; well, mostly taking things apart in all sorts of places – in the garage, the back yard and down by the river.
>
> Some days we would just sit there and watch insects. But mostly we were climbing trees, challenging ourselves. I remember working with the fast flowing river discovering how to have fun without drowning. I didn't know it at the time, but we were developing social skills – working with each other, getting along and sorting out our differences – who was going to lead the next game.
>
> We used to make up a lot of games. We began to see other people's skills – Joey was very good at seeing things intuitively, and Billy could fix things in his dad's tool shed – we relied on him for many engineering projects. We developed trust in each other; we were in real situations where you had to count on people. We were looking at birds squawking at each other, all the life in the wetlands, watching the fish and their cycles. You learn a lot about life cycles watching salmon – see them spawning, and watching them die. Without making a big deal of it, we were connecting with the impermanence of life, the changing of the seasons, and how things are.

My wife and I both work hard. We put in long hours — virtually all inside — and it is a struggle just to keep the kids fed, dressed and schooled. But I see that there are so many times in the day where we are making choices that involve sitting in front of a computer, TV or video screen.

Inspired by *Wireless Radiation Rescue,* we decided to make an effort to wean ourselves off of these entertainments. It seemed daunting at first. The kids rebelled. Then my wife and I sat down and had a family discussion about how all these technology things had been part of making me sick. They, of course, shot back that was because I was 'old' and they were just kids so it was okay for them. I didn't subject them to all the evidence, but my wife and I did our best to explain why spending too much time around these electronics was not a good idea for kids.

We found that rather than trying to tackle this head-on, that we would plan some outings. As I unplugged more myself, I got better — I was sleeping much better and

had more energy. So instead of collapsing in front of the TV when I got home, I'd say 'let's go outside and kick a ball around'.

Once we were outside more, I noticed the kids were really into it and even took themselves outside now and then. Our somewhat pasty-looking kids began to look healthier. Sometimes we just go outside and sit on the ground and chat. And listen to each other.

What Was It Like When You Were Young?

What kind of stories are the children you know going to tell? What stories, and values, are they going to pass along to their children, and grandchildren? If the rate of technology continues at the current supersonic speed what kind of lives are all of us going to have in ten years? In twenty? It's not too late. We can take better care of the health of our families, and our home – this blue planet is our only home.

From Good Intentions to Effective Changes

This is a lot of information; important things for us to consider to safeguard our families. The challenge: not to get overwhelmed and give up into hopelessness. After you waded through Strategy 3, I included an intention plan to help focus on what you wanted to deal with first – your priorities. Here is that list again. Just skip over it, if you want.

Reviewing Our Radiation Rescue Intentions

Top Priorities – what I want to tackle first:

Secondary priorities – what I want to deal with after that:

I should consult a professional to assess the following:

Other environmental exposures I want to address:

Now that you have been through Strategy 4, which has enough aspirations to last a lifetime, let's look again at winnowing this down into bite size chunks.

Our Radiation Rescue Action Plan

Area	Action intended	Action completed
Front Porch		
Master Bedroom		
Children's Rooms		
Bathroom		
Kitchen		
Laundry Room		
Vacuum Cleaner		
Office		
Cordless Phones		

Area	Action intended	Action completed
Internet Access		
Other Environmental Exposures		
Your Physical Health		
Nutritional Supplementation		
Dental Health		
Other Well Being/Lifestyle Factors		
RR Family Communication Challenge		
RR Safer-Tech Family Challenge		
Other Personal Goals		

WE CAN MEET THIS CHALLENGE but please don't imagine that you are going to reduce the risks all at once.

We have been developing this unsafe-tech environment for a long time and many people are deeply hooked. Detoxing from a digital addiction

Hope For the Future

may become the latest trend.

Let's just take this one step at a time, and feel good about each exposure we reduce. If you have got this far in the book, you have already accomplished a lot!

You now know more about this issue than most of the regulators and legislators setting and approving the safety limits.

I hope you will continue through this last chapter to hear from some of our experts about their hopes for the future, while you contemplate yours, for you and your loved ones.

See Hope For the Future for more details.

Hope For the Future

Moving from Knowledge to Action

It may surprise you to know (or maybe by now it won't surprise you) that some American scientists have been telling their government about EMR biological effects for more than 35 years!

Robert O. Becker, MD, was one of the researchers looking into the U.S. navy's plans to install a 6,000 mile underwater messaging system to communicate with submarines.

Dr. Becker said:

> As far as I know, our testimony (in 1975) was the first ever openly given by American scientists stating that electromagnetic energy had health effects in doses below those needed to heat tissue, and that power lines might therefore be hazardous to human health.

We criticized the White House Office of Telecommunications Policy for failing to follow up a tentative 1971 warning that harmful effects from electro-pollution were proven.

There are hopes that the US administration will take a courageous stand on this issue.

As I mentioned early on, one of the leading lights in fighting the installation of cell towers is Eileen O'Connor, the founder of EM Radiation Research in the UK. She was one of the presenters to the 2010 President's Cancer Panel that studied the possible links between radiation (nuclear and electro-magnetic) and cancer.

Ms. O'Connor was pleased the issue is being taken seriously:

> President Obama has said science is about ensuring that facts and evidence are never twisted or obscured by politics or ideology. It's about listening to what our scientists have to say, even when it's inconvenient and I welcome this approach.

Many of us have the "audacity of hope" that this administration, and the next one, will show true leadership in this other inconvenient truth. Steps taken to protect people's health are likely to be echoed around the world.

As you may know, most politicians take their lead from the majority of the electorate's demands; it's not the other way around. Yes, there's industry lobbying, but when enough of us unite to demand safer limits for this technology for the health of all of us, especially our children, then things will change.

What Your Town Can Do

Have some shiny new palm trees, pine trees or church spires sprung up in your neighborhood? Near your child's school? You can do something about these cell tower antennas.

There is an excellent book edited by B. Blake Levitt: *Cell Towers: Wireless Convenience? or Environmental Hazard?* This is a quote from Blake Levitt:

Something municipalities fail to keep in mind is the basic legal fact that it is up to the providers of a service or product to prove that their wares are safe. It is not up to us to prove that they are unsafe. The tele-communications industry has largely failed to do that. Just because they are within the FCC guidelines for RF emission, does not prove safety. No town today should allow itself to be intimidated by telecom service providers or adjunct industries like tower companies...

Those in decision-making positions need to understand that this form of land use regulation is very different than traditional forms. This is NOT just an aesthetic issue. It is a medical one.

This could be used at a public meeting. Most likely, no official would sign. Their reluctance, however, should be of interest to those residents, parents, and others who will be directly affected.

Statement of Accountability

My stated position is that the (cell tower antenna, Wi-Fi router, Smart Meter) that has been proposed or approved in or near (_____) should go ahead or remain as it does not present significant health risks within _____ *(feet or meters.)*

I am aware that the World Health Organization has reclassified this radiation and cautioned "it is possibly carcinogenic to human health," and that adverse biological effects have been linked with the levels of radiation emitted by this technology, including increased cancer and leukemia with proximity to cell tower antennas, and of other health risks with wireless exposures. I am aware of the research indicating children and pregnant women are most vulnerable; that many countries have set limits on the placement of this technology; and that cancer and other related diseases can take years to develop.

I acknowledge that public health official David Carpenter, MD called government regulators, "Just plain wrong" and their standards are challenged by many other experts as not accurate, and not protecting us. I am aware these regulations did *not* consider adverse effects on children, nor long-term exposure. I have heard this statement to the wireless industry by Dr. David Gee, of the BioInitiative Report:

> They are forewarned now, and saying 'but we were in compliance with ICNIRP (the international regulatory agency) safety limits' will not be sufficient reason for ignoring the growing evidence.

And I have read the remarks by electrical engineer Alasdair Philips:

> Many people living near masts (cell tower antennas), and other RF exposures, experience ill health: sleep disruption, headaches, dizziness, behaviour changes in children, nosebleeds, epilepsy, and increased rates of cancer. (See www.powerwatch.org.uk)

I have heard the quote by cardiologist Stephen Sinatra, MD that "Electro-pollution is the greatest medical threat of our time. As the heart is electrical in nature and vulnerable to this radiation, there can be cardiac, as well as cancer, risks from these exposures. Pregnant women, children, and those with heart disease are most at risk."

If you have been assured by another expert in this field that this system does not present health risks, please list his or her name and credentials: _____

The reason I believe this installation be implemented or remain is: _____

I believe that those responsible for this installation _____ do not have any past or present health-related disputes regarding this technology.

Please note exceptions: _____

I believe that any adverse health effects, or medical conditions, attributed to this short and long-term exposure are covered by the insurance policy provided by _____

Your name: (*Please print*)_____

Your title and official position:

_____

Today's date: _____

Your signature: _____

Witnessed by: _____

For your information, a list of the individuals who have been sent this letter has been forwarded to _____
(media names). As there is strong community interest in this issue, they have been sent a copy of this letter and asked to follow up with you.

(This form is available to download at: www.radiationrescue.org)

Professor Johansson is widely regarded as one of the leading experts. When officials, at all levels, heed his words we will all be more hopeful for the future:

> I strongly advise all governments to take the issue of electromagnetic health hazards seriously and to take action while there is still time.
>
> Governments should act decisively to protect public health by changing the exposure standards to be biologically-based, communicating the results of the independent science on this topic and aggressively researching links with a multitude of associated medical conditions.

As you know, there are many things we aspire to in this life. Fundamentally, is there anything more truly worthwhile than safeguarding our family and the future of our children?

That's why I have spent more than four years researching and writing this book. For you, and for your family.

Promising Signs On the Horizon

Are you old enough to remember the movie The Graduate? A young man is given a tip for success by one of his parents' friends, "The future, Benjamin, is plastics." The advice now might be: fiber optics. Why? Several of our experts have mentioned this as the wave of the future.

Progress In Technology

Fiber Optics – Safe and Secure

Many telecom technical experts also prefer this system. One told me that, "Fiber optic lines are thin strands of optically pure glass. This is the best way to move large amounts of data – digital information – over long distances. Security is a big factor, (as we mentioned before). Fiber optics is a secure, closed system (the shot-gun approach of satellites and wireless radiation firing through space is not). And fiber optics do not have the same radiation issues."

Evidently, there are plans to bring fiber optic connections to homes and businesses, instead of wireless, for our Internet access.

Let's promote this! The safest communities will provide this now essential online access with fiber optics to buildings that provide cable/wired access.

Not everyone in the wireless industry is onside. Not yet.

Breaking Out of the Cyber Cocoon

If you have read through most of this book – glanced at a few pages? – you know this message is piercing.

It cuts to the heart of our techno-addictions: have we become too attached to the convenience and to those scintillating 'pings' and downloaded rings of cyber-connections? Are we immersing ourselves in clouds of radiation in the process? Are we closeting ourselves, and our children, inside and filling space with hyper-speed entertainment, the instant gratification of texting and Twittering?

Acknowledging any addiction is a tough message to take in. And that's without all of the "too scary" stuff about cancer and brain damage.

I have tried my best, without sugar-coating anything, to focus on the ways we can turn around this potentially perilous situation, and reduce the health risks, without losing the conveniences of this never-ending stream of technology.

Now, let's rouse our energies and look on the bright side of possibilities and prevention. Working together, let's do what we can to rescue our families. I am hopeful.

As a whole generation of baby boomers age – many who are already self-proclaimed 'crackberry' addicts – there is concern about health effects after so many years of sitting in front of computers and being hooked on electronics.

It is encouraging that there are treatments evolving to deal with these effects.

Clinical Progress

There is hope on the clinical horizon. Innovative doctors are working on effective ways to heal, and prevent, symptoms and conditions related to EMR exposure.

There is also hope for the millions of people already suffering from electro-sensitivity, and for those with Autism Spectrum symptoms and related neurological conditions.

Let's demand more research in this area as the conventional medical approach of relying mainly on X-ray diagnostic tests, pharmaceuticals and/or surgery does not seem the best approach when dealing with the environmental assaults which we have been discussing.

It seems we need a multi-disciplinary approach focusing on holistic, non-invasive ways to heal and prevent environmental conditions. And, as the electromagnetic fields affect us on a frequency level, we should be looking at energy medicine for some of the clinical clues.

I am going to continue calling upon our clinical and research experts, and others, to give us the information and tools we need to safeguard our health.

Parents and Grandparents Demanding Safer Products

I am confident that most people will follow the lead of our library mum and make an effort to cut back on cell phone use and get our families unplugged and outside whenever we can, and that informed parents, grandparents and educators will limit our children's exposure in the ways we have discussed.

As we have seen in Europe, some legislators are listening to the independent scientists and inching forward to bring regulations within recommended safe limits, and safer products, including a less hazardous baby monitor, are being developed. All are encouraging steps. Will all of this be in time to prevent the global EMR-related pandemic that some fear? Can we rescue this hyper-tech generation? Yes, if we act now.

Progress With Our Families' Safer-Tech Challenge

Library Mum

Basically, this program has made me more aware of the addiction that my family and I have nurtured around technology. I will be increasingly more wary of gadgets which promise to increase my well being by providing me with efficiency tools.

In his video series, John Bradshaw uses the metaphor of a hanging mobile to show that when one part of the mobile moves and changes, it sends reverberations and changes throughout the whole system. I feel that this book has done a similar thing with our family. It seems that the changes that I am attempting to implement are leading to profound changes in our family interactions in general. It hasn't all been easy... at times.

On one hand, these changes have been bringing tensions to the surface (for example, my son's Internet and technology savvy seem to be in direct conflict with my desire for a low radiation home and a de-emphasis on 'screen culture').

So, through these changes, we are learning how to navigate each other's needs and respect each other; whereas without this particular technology challenge, we have had very little conflict to work through (I found myself at the height of frustration yesterday when I thought that my son was reconnecting the Wi-Fi and I pulled the computer power cord out of the outlet and banned the computer from use!)

The changes that I've been making have also had an impact on my relationship with myself. The cell phone, in particular, makes me feel important and necessary; efficient, productive and connected.

This is a heady mixture in a society that places such value on these qualities. The cell phone is a transformative wand which takes me from being a 'housewife' and 'mother' (negative terms in today's society) and magically transforms me into a 'modern, West Coast, work-at-home executive.'

Is this true? Is it what I really feel and think about – or is it the effective machinations of savvy marketers?

Because every change invokes a challenge to a personal relationship, my attempts to cut down the electromagnetic radiation in our lives are not simply a matter of just making simple technology changes.

For this reason, I have experienced profound shifts. All this navigating takes personal energy.

And so, I have not been able to implement all of the book's suggestions in a straightforward, progressive way.

Instead, the process looks messy – it has turnarounds and circle-backs. This will likely continue. Yet, as I reflect on this today, I believe that this is natural.

Even blame, self-doubt, perfectionism and discouragement can be seen as part of a larger spiritual process of growth and renewal (as long as they don't lead to an abandonment of the whole project!).

We begin to exercise our right to make choices and to create an environment rather than accepting one that is pre-packaged. This, in itself, is sufficient reason to begin the journey!

Neighbor Dad

Changing gears is not as easy as it may sound. Some days, I feel we have failed hopelessly with our good intentions to live a more simple life, and to rely less on all this technology. The least bit of rain keeps the kids inside and begging for their gaming.

My wife still goes right to the computer in her jammies, bleary-eyed and clutching her coffee mug, to check her email. We have made some progress since reading this book. We should feel good about that, but this is going to take some time. I'm determined, though, to ease us gently away from this fixation, and focus on the successes, and more family fun, which we are enjoying these days.

Your Action Plan

As you can see, this is a process with "turnarounds and circle-backs". As these families have described, we are not only dealing with our own households, we are dealing with a culture that has evolved around instant gratification. Please take it step by step, feel good about every exposure you reduce, and don't give up.

Your Safer-Tech Family Challenge?

When you are ready, see if you can get everyone on board and make this a sporting event. Try a positive approach: add more of the outdoor activities that your family enjoys, rather than ripping the gaming stations out of the kids' hands. And, please be patient, with your family, and yourself.

Each week, spend one evening away from the computers and the TV's, and get outside for a walk in your neighborhood, or a nearby park. Try "no-screens" for a day. Or a week?

Check out garage sales for good deals on bikes, balls, badminton racquets, playing cards and board games. Ask everyone in your family, depending on his or her age, to come up with a non-electronic activity for that week. Maybe it's a rousing game of cards, or charades?

I know we are really busy, and many of our children have back-to-back lessons, sports and other after-school activities. These too can contribute to limiting EMR exposure, particularly if we watch the soccer game instead of texting on the sidelines.

I read one local hockey arena went wireless so the parents could work on their laptops during those long games and practices. How often do you see families at a park, or on the beach, and instead of being together, instead of really being there, they are immersed in the virtual world? What does this teach our children about how to interact in the real world?

Once you go through the withdrawal and your texting, gaming, Twittering fingers stop shaking, you may find you feel greatly invigorated by safer-tech activities.

This technology, and the world-wide Internet, have brought our global village many benefits. We can continue to enjoy and expand upon those. As with most powerful influences, we just need to use them more wisely.

Progress In Consumer Awareness

The message is getting out. People are waking up. Remember that great line from the film Network? "We're mad as hell and we aren't going to take it anymore."

Dr. McKinney has offered to work with me to develop awareness and education and programs to get this message out:

> As results surface from scientists, researchers and clinicians it becomes important to share this information with citizens around the globe.

We will keep this updated on our website. And will continue to bring you the latest research and technical advice.

We owe a debt of gratitude to the many people who helped with this book and to the thousands more working tirelessly in this field.

Recently, I wrote to one of our contributors:

> Thanks to the dedication of pioneers like yourself, I predict we are reaching a tipping point where consumers, particularly parents and grandparents, are waking up. Soon the industry is not going to be able to hold back the tide of public demand for the truth, for truly safe products. And governments will be pressured into action for accurate safe standards.

I have asked some of our contributors for their hopes for the future.

Dr. William Rea, and several others, offered that they were optimistic. This is encouraging as Dr. Rea, for example, is treating people every day who are already suffering from EMR exposure.

Dr. Stephen Sinatra:

> Educating physicians, other health professionals, and the public is key to meeting the health challenges of electro-pollution – the greatest medical hazard today.

> First, increased medical awareness will assist in the diagnosis and treatment of those presenting with related symptoms – dizziness, sleep disruption, tinnitus, and heart rate and rhythm disturbances. People will get the treatment they need, and may avoid tests (often involving diagnostic radiation exposure) and pharmacologic intervention (often involving side effects.) Second, education will raise public awareness about the need to use wired and wireless electronic devices with more caution and could encourage legislators to bring the safety standards in line with the science.

Alasdair Philips:

My hope for the future is that politicians and business leaders start acting with integrity regarding sustainable living and deal with problems like EMF/RF exposure now instead of ignoring them in order to make short-term financial gains.

Dr. Magda Havas:

I hope that those individuals who are in positions of authority, and this includes parents, teachers, employers, as well as government officials, will make the necessary changes required to minimize our exposure to electromagnetic pollution. I hope that it will not take decades, as it did with tobacco, to do the right thing. May those who are sensitive, who are the 'early warning indicators', not suffer in vain. May their experience alert us to the problem and give us the courage to resolve it. May we have the wisdom to live up to our name Homo sapien sapien and not have to change it to Homo greedicus ignoramus.

Dr. Sarah Starkey:

My hope for the future is that people will come to accept that creating a sustainable future for our planet involves reducing artificial electromagnetic fields. I would like children to grow up knowing that to protect their own health, that of future generations and their environment they need to limit their use of microwave-emitting technologies.

Dr. Heather McKinney:

My hope is that consumers around the world will raise their voices to encourage scientists, politicians, and corporate executives to be proactive, and look at this situation as an opportunity for research and long term restructuring. I am optimistic that this can happen.

Dr. Carrie Hyman:

We need more private citizens asking questions about the safety of these products. We all need to work hand in hand with clinicians, environmentalists and politicians to address this health issue quickly and responsibly.

Dr. Louis Slesin:

My hope is some breaking down of the research roadblocks. This is a challenge as there are so many vested interests on the hazards side; so much money involved. To be honest, I am not optimistic. I am encouraged, however, on the clinical side; there's progress with biomedical applications – this may be the key.

Dr. Devra Davis:

The government should work with phone companies to protect our children and to provide data to Professor Gandhi, and to other independent researchers, so that we can find the safest way to use this revolutionary technology which has also brought many benefits. In an ideal world, the profitable companies would compete to design the safest and sleekest phones.

Now You've Heard The Whole Story

How are you feeling about all this now? Not too overwhelmed? I am confident in speaking for our contributors: our hope for you is the ability to make more informed decisions, and to use wired and wireless technology more safely.

We are also working to increase medical awareness so you can have more support from your doctor and others charged with the public wellbeing. And we're fighting hard to make our schools safer for all.

To summarize, let's take a look at these strategies again.

7 Key Reminders – wired over wireless and corded over cordless.

1. Switch your cordless phones to corded ones. Please don't give up your landline phone (and they are also health-savvy gifts);

2. Seek wired solutions for all things wireless, including your Internet access, keep laptops and all wireless devices off your lap, and <u>please do not use digital baby monitors, or wireless sensor pads</u>;

3. Keep your cell phone simple (basic, low SAR), and away from your head, your heart, pregnant women and the young. Limit it's use;

4. Use your mobile's speakerphone, rather than wireless, or wired headsets, and remember the most hazardous option of all is holding a mobile device against your head;

5. Avoid using a cell phone for an alarm clock, or sleeping near it;

6. Tell your airline and hotel that you want a wireless-free environment;

7. Talk to your local legislators, calmly and clearly. Provide some information (not overwhelming them) and ask for a response.

Please take this slowly and don't lose heart about the future. We can meet this challenge. We just need to keep focused and keep going. It's a journey that will bring many benefits. Ready to give it a try?

May you rediscover the delights of unplugging and stepping outside of your electronic cocoon, and reconnecting with the natural world.

May you have the courage to face the inconvenient truths, for yourself and your family, and this blue planet – our only home.

May you, and all of our children, and grandchildren, thrive.

And, after reading (skimming?) this book, I hope you are inspired by our risk reduction plan for optimal health. This whole book, and our strategies, can also be a vital part of your anti-aging program, addressing the key factors that most other approaches are missing. Longevity is not only living longer, but living well – healthy aging in this new digital age.

> *You will succeed if you persevere; and you will find a joy in overcoming obstacles. I have confidence in the human spirit.*
>
> Helen Keller

> *Never doubt the ability of a small group of thoughtful people to change the world. Indeed, it is the only thing that ever has.*
>
> Margaret Mead

Resources

Research, Advocacy and Electro-Sensitivity Support Groups

USA

• **www.antennafreeunion.org**

The San Francisco Neighborhood Antenna-Free Union (SNAFU) is a grass-roots, city-wide coalition of individual residents and neighborhood organizations.

• **www.bioinitiative.org**

In 2007, an international working group of scientists, researchers and public health policy professionals (The BioInitiative Working Group) released its report on electromagnetic fields (EMF) and health.

• **www.electromagnetichealth.org**

One of the most effective voices is that of Camilla Rees. She is the founder of ElectromagneticHealth.org and co-author with Dr. Magda Havas of the book, *Public Health SOS: The Shadow Side of the Wireless Revolution.*

• **www.emrpolicy.org**

The mission of The EMR Policy Institute is to foster a better understanding of the environmental and human biological effects from such exposures.

• **www.energyfields.org**

The Council on Wireless Technology Impacts is concerned about the safe use of technologies which use electromagnetic radiation.

• **www.ewg.org**

Environmental Working Group (EWG), a Washington, DC-based nonprofit organization, is dedicated to protecting children, babies, and infants in the womb from health problems attributed to a wide array of toxic contaminants. Their other mission is the relevant federal policies.

• **www.guineapigsrus.org**

Joanne Mueller's pamphlet, *Are You A Guinea Pig?* tells how to sleep better and feel better by reducing EMR exposure.

• **www.microwavenews.com**

Microwave News is meticulously researched and documented, making it one of the world's most authoritative sources of information on EMR/EMF health risks. Its founder, and editor, Dr. Louis Slesin, has worked tirelessly on this issue for nearly 30 years.

• **www.centerforsaferwireless.org**

Christine Hoch founded Center For Safer Wireless, a national non-profit organization dedicated to enhancing the public's understanding of wireless product safety, especially cautioning parents about children's use of cell phones. Based in Virginia, the group engages in educational activities aimed at increasing awareness of radio-frequency radiation, electromagnetic radiation, and the potential health implications of wireless products and technology.

CANADA

• **www.causetm.ca**

Citizens Against Un-safe Emissions (CAUSE) was founded by Sharon Noble. Her group has made great strides forward in educating the public and their Council of Colwood, BC. The Mayor signed the Porto Alegre Resolution – a first in North America, and recognized electro-sensitivity – a first in Canada.

• **www.citizensforsafetechnology.org**

Founded by Una St Clair-Moniz, Citizens for Safe Technology successfully educated their council in White Rock, BC, who passed a motion to ask the Canadian Federal Government to review the Safety Code 6 standards that regulate wireless technologies. They have also focused on school boards.

• **www.hans.org**

The Health Action Network is a charitable natural health resource. HANS provides information through its website and regular events.

• www.weepinitiative.org

The Canadian Initiative to Stop Wireless, Electric, and Electromagnetic Pollution (WEEP) has a mission to inform the public about the potential environmental effects associated with electromagnetic immersions.

IRELAND

• www.ideaireland.org

The Irish Doctors' Environmental Association (IDEA) was established by health professionals to promote the right to health worldwide.

UK

• www.es-uk.info

Sarah Dacre is a trustee of ES-UK. This is a registered charity in the UK advising and educating about electro-sensitivity, its possible triggers and ways to lessen symptoms.

• www.mastsanity.org

Mast Sanity is a national group of community members who campaign against the unsafe placement of mobile communications towers.

• www.mast-victims.org

This is an international community website for people suffering adverse health effects from mobile phone masts in the vicinity of their homes.

• www.powerwatch.org.uk

Powerwatch is a non-profit independent organization that has been studying the health effects of electro-magnetic fields for the last 20 years, and provides information to help the public understand this complex issue.

• www.radiationresearch.org

EM Radiation Research Trust researches EMR and related health effects; has a leaflet called *Precautionary Approach to Wireless Communication;* lobbies the U.K. Government and the E.U. for policy change based on proven science.

• **www.wifiinschools.org.uk**

Wi-Fi In Schools has been set up by Dr. Sarah Starkey and a small group of other scientists concerned about the rapid spread of wireless technologies in schools. The group recommends application of the precautionary principle.

• **www.wiredchild.org**

WiredChild is a charity run by a group of concerned parents, raising awareness of the potential risks to children of exposure to radiation from mobile phones and other wireless technology.

EUROPE:

• **www.hese-project.org (German)**
• **www.hese-project.org/hese-uk (English)**

HESE (Human Ecological Social Economical project) is an international, interdisciplinary collaboration of scientists, institutions and informed lay people, which brings together research and advocacy information in several languages. Many of its contributors have suffered health effects from EMR.

• **www.next-up.org**

This France-based organization brings together the latest research, regulations and European news on lobbying efforts and public action.

• **www.priartem.fr**

PRIARTéM (Pour une réglementation des Implantations d'Antennes Relais de Téléphonie Mobile) is a citizens' group created in 2000 to monitor the installation of mobile phone antennas.

AUSTRALIA:

• **www.emfacts.com**

EMFacts was established in 1997 by Don Maisch, PhD as an independent source of information on the possible health and safety issues arising from human exposure to EMR.

• **www.emraustralia.com.au**

EMR Australia is a consumer advocacy group which is working to alert people about the growing concerns in that country.

NEW ZEALAND:

• **www.neilcherry.com**

Dr. Neil Cherry (1946-2003) was Associate Professor of Environmental Health at Lincoln University. He had discussions with many of the researchers.

• **www.canterbury.cyberplace.co.nz/ouruhia**

Oururah NZ is a group providing information on its website about cell tower antennas - masts - and mobile phone health hazards.

• **www.banthetower.co.nz**

Ban The Tower is working hard to alert people to the risks of wireless radiation and where cell towers are located, and planned.

INTERNATIONAL:

• **www.doctorsforsaferschools.org**

This international advisory board is an association of professionals, and others, concerned about the health risks of EMR, especially wireless radiation exposure, in schools. The mission is to give parents, educators, doctors and others accurate information on health concerns and the safer-tech solutions.

• **www.iemfa.org**

The International Electro-Magnetic Fields Alliance is an independent global body of empirically-based scientific experts, with a multidisciplinary health focus. Founding members: Alex Swinkels, Netherlands; Brian Stein, Eileen O'Connor, United Kingdom; Camilla Rees, Diana Warren, Elizabeth Barris, Elizabeth Kelley, Janet Newton, United States; Daniel Oberhausen, France; Don Maisch, Australia; Sissel Halmøy, Norway

• **www.icems.eu**

The International Commission for Electromagnetic Safety (ICEMS) is a non-profit organization registered in Italy that promotes research and develops strategies for assessment, prevention, management and communication.

• **EMF Refugees: The International Coalition for an Electromagnetic Safe Planet (IC-ESP)** This group was founded by Paul Doyon, MA to bring people together to form their own EMF-free communities in natural environments where they can heal and create healing environments for the Earth and others. They have an excellent flyer on ES, *Unwittingly Affected.*

Autism Related Issues

• **www.generationrescue.org**

Generation Rescue is an international movement of scientists and physicians researching the causes and treatments for autism, ADHD and chronic illness, while parent volunteers mentor thousands of families in recovering their children.

• **www.thriiive.com**

THRiiiVE!!! was founded by Dana Gorman. Their mission is to sort through the plethora of information available from all disciplines that impact health, organize it and disseminate it in a useful format so everyone can make informed choices that are beneficial to themselves and their family. She also brings together leading researchers and clinicians dealing with Autism Spectrum Disorders, and other neurological conditions.

Children & Nature

• **www.childrenandnature.org**

The Children & Nature Network (C&NN) was created to encourage and support the people and organizations working to reconnect children with nature. C&NN provides access to the latest news and research in the field and a peer-to-peer network of researchers and individuals, educators and organizations dedicated to children's health and wellbeing.

• **www.childnature.ca**

In North America there is a growing movement to reconnect children and families to nature for improved health and wellbeing. The Child and Nature Alliance is a non-profit organization in British Columbia that is formalizing the movement provincially, and eventually across Canada.

Medical Clinics/Professional Practices

Robert Abell, ND, LAc is a naturopathic physician who uses auricular medicine, homeopathy, acupuncture and Biotherapeutic Drainage as his primary therapeutic tools. He lectures on the assessment and treatments of neurological disorders including ADHD and autism. Dr. Abell treats children with ADHD and autism in his clinics and does phone consultations.

Be Well Acupuncture & Natural Medicine Clinic
Laguna Hills, California & Austin, Texas
Website: **www.bewellhealthclinic.com**

Nancy A. Didriksen, PhD has a private practice in health psychology/behavior medicine and neuropsychology. She specializes in evaluation and treatment, including for EMF sensitivities. She is an adjunct professor of psychology at the University of North Texas.

Richardson, TX
Email: **drnancy@airmail.net**

Leslie S. Feinberg, DC developed NeuroModulation Technique as a result of his many years of studying energetic medicine and the principles of western science and Traditional Chinese Medicine. Dr. Feinberg teaches this technique to other health professionals from many disciplines.

Columbia Chiropractic Clinic
NeuroModulation Technique NMT Seminars,
Hermiston, Oregon USA
Website: **www.nmt.md**

Mark Hyman, MD and Elizabeth Boham, MD practice at the UltraWellness Center where they focus on identifying and treating the underlying causes of illness, starting with extensive diagnostic testing. Dr. Mark Hyman is the author of several books on wellness issues including: environmental influences, supplementation, metabolism, detoxification and the conditions ADHD and autism. Dr. Hyman also offers training programs for health professionals through the Institute for Functional Medicine.

Lenox, MA
Email: office@ultrawellnesscenter.com
Website: **www.drhyman.com**

Carrie Hyman, LAc, OMD is available for speaking engagements. Topics include: "Maintaining Health In The Wireless Age"; "Cell Phones, Kids & Us: The Inconvenient Truth About Convenient Technology" and "You Can't Fool Mother Nature: EMF & the Environment."

Contact: **dochyman1@gmail.com**

Dietrich Klinghardt, MD, PhD was one of the first practitioners in the U.S. to include aggressive detoxification in his medical treatment strategies. He has pioneered many diagnostic and detoxification strategies and is considered one of the worldwide leading authorities in this rapidly advancing field. There is an extensive list on the following website, under Referrals, of practitioners who have trained with Dr. Klinghardt.

Klinghardt Academy of Neurobiology
Website: **www.klinghardt.org**

Stephanie McCarter, MD is an internal medicine/environmental medicine physician who works alongside Dr. Rea, treating those with EMF sensitivities. She is also active in bringing together physicians, healthcare professionals, researchers, and scientists to explore this biochemical phenomenon.

Website: **www.ehcd.com**

Jean Monro, MD is the Medical Director at the Breakspear Medical Group in England, and is a London Hospital Medical School trained physician. She is internationally active in educating other physicians, colleagues, patients, and the public about physiological mechanisms behind EMF sensitivity, and possible treatments.

Breakspear Medical Group
Herts, UK
Website: **www.breakspearmedical.com**

Ron Overberg, PhD, CCN, RD, LD is a nutritionist at the EHC-D. One of his specialties at the clinic is working with EMF sensitive patients. He is also active in helping to educate physicians and the public about EMF sensitivity, and corresponding nutrition considerations.

Website: **www.ehcd.com**

Thomas Rau, MD is the medical director of the Paracelsus Klinik in Switzerland which is the core of the international network of Paracelsus Biological Medicine. It was established in 1958 and is widely recognized as a center of excellence for natural medicine.

Website: **www.drrau.com**

William J. Rea, MD is a thoracic and cardiovascular surgeon with a strong passion for the environmental aspects of health and disease. Dr. Rea is founder of The Environmental Health Center - Dallas, Texas, which offers comprehensive medical tests and treats human health problems including sensitivities to pollens, molds, dust, foods, chemicals, air (indoor/outdoor), water, electrical sensitivity (electromagnetic- EMF) and many more.

Website: **www.ehcd.com**

Gay Riley, MS, RD, CCN, NASM-CPT is a licensed and registered dietitian able to provide Medical Nutrition Therapy (MNT), and a Certified Clinical Nutritionist, which includes training in complementary alternative modalities, therapeutic supplementation, diagnostic testing and functional nutrition, and education in therapeutic applications for vitamin and mineral supplementation.

Richardson, TX
Website: **www.netnutritionist.com**

Sanoviv Medical Institute, founded by Dr. Myron Wentz, is a cutting edge medical and healing center, located south of San Diego, in Baja California. Sanoviv offers integrative, patient-centered medical treatments complemented by individualized personal care programs.

Website: **www.sanoviv.com**

Hans-Christoph Scheiner, MD has been practicing holistic medicine in Munich, Germany, since 1975 with a focus on natural healing and psychotherapy. Dr. Scheiner is an author and presents medical expert opinions at parliamentary hearings. Dr. Scheiner's book, written with Ana Scheiner, is *Mobilfunk – die verkaufte Gesundheit*, 2006.

Institut für Holistische Medizin - München
Website: **www.drscheiner-muenchen.de**

Stephen T. Sinatra, MD, FACC, FACN, CNS is a board-certified cardiologist, certified bioenergetic psychotherapist and certified nutrition and anti-aging specialist. He is a fellow in the American College of Cardiology and the American College of Nutrition, former chief of cardiology at Manchester Memorial Hospital, and an assistant clinical professor of medicine at the University of Connecticut School of Medicine. He writes a monthly national newsletter entitled Heart, Health and Nutrition (Healthy Directions, L.L.C.), lectures world-wide, and facilitates health-related workshops.

Website: **www.heartmdinstitute.com**

Dr. Briana Sinatra ND, LAc, MSA and Dr. Drew Sinatra ND, LAc, MSA utilize a holistic approach to reduce the detrimental effects radiation can have on a cellular, biochemical and physiologic level. This includes education on ways to identify and reduce EMR exposure, along with ways to help the body cope with unavoidable EMR. Dr. Briana Sinatra uses Traditional Chinese Medicine and Dr. Drew Sinatra practices 5-Element Acupuncture to help connect people to the cycles of nature, which are disrupted with EMR exposure.

Living Wellness Center, South Surrey, British Columbia
Website: **www.livingwellness.ca**

Martha Stark, MD is a Harvard trained physician. She has a private practice in psychoanalysis, and is on faculty at Harvard Medical School in the Center for Psychoanalytic Studies. She works with environmental physicians and scientists to explore the impact of physiological EMFs on the body, including oxidative stress, excitotoxicity, and mitochondrial disruption.

Harvard Medical School
Email: **MarthaStarkMD@HMS.harvard.edu**

Jacob Teitelbaum, MD is a board-certified internist and Medical Director of the national Fibromyalgia and Fatigue Centers, Inc., in the U.S. He focuses on expanding the understanding of hypothalamic dysfunction in Fibromyalgia (FMS) and Chronic Fatigue Syndrome (CFIDS). His work has led to the development of an effective treatment protocol for these diseases.

Website: **www.endfatigue.com**

To Find a Practitioner of Holistic/Complementary Medicine

Website: **www.holisticmedicine.org**

Research and Education

Magda Havas, PhD is an associate professor at Trent University. She focuses on teaching and leading research on the health and environmental effects of chemical contaminants on electromagnetic pollution.

Environmental & Resource Studies, Trent University
Peterborough, ON Canada

Heather McKinney, PhD is a researcher who specializes in strategic planning for effective change and health improvement within individuals, organizations and communities. She is working with the author in developing the Wireless Radiation Rescue education program.

Email: **DrHeatherMcKinney@gmail.com**

Cyril W. Smith, PhD is a physicist and author. He has a special interest in the scientific mechanism of EHS and aims to help healthcare professionals understand the quantum science behind this phenomenon.

Eccles, Manchester UK

Biological Dentists

International Association of Mercury Free Dentists
Website: **www.dentalwellness4u.com**

International Association of Biological Dentistry and Medicine
Website: **www.iabdm.org**

Holistic Dental Association
Website: **www.holisticdental.org**

Professional Services

Healthy Buildings:

International Institute for Bau-Biologie (IBE)
Website: **www.buildingbiology.net**

IBE/IBN Certified Consultants:

CANADA

Morriston, Ontario
Safe Living Technologies Inc.
Rob Metzinger, President
Testing equipment and protective/solution products, including
shielding materials and air tube headsets.
Email: metzinger@safelivingtechnologies.ca
Website: **www.safelivingtechnologies.ca**

Montreal, Quebec
3E Electro-magnetic Environmental Expertise Inc.
Stéphane Belainsky
Website: **www.em3e.com**

Victoria, British Columbia
Rainbow Consulting
Katharina Gustavs, Building Biology Environmental Consultant (IBN)
Website: **www.buildingbiology.ca**

USA

Carlsbad, California
Environmental Testing & Technology, Inc.(ET&T)
ET&T was founded in 1986 by Peter Sierck to provide an indoor
environmental testing and consulting service for patients, physicians,
home owners, corporations, institutions and builders.
Website: **www.emfrf.com**

San Diego, California
Gust Environmental
Larry Gust
Email: lgust@wavecable.com
Website: **www.healbuildings.com**

New York City, Long Island, Eastern NJ, CT, lower and upper state NY
Matt Waletzke, BBEC
Healthy Dwellings Tel: 612.242.4558
Email: matt@healthydwellings.com
Website: **www.healthydwellings.com**

Clearwater, Florida
Indoor Environmental Technologies, Inc.
William H. Spates, III – BBEI
Website: **www.ietbuildinghealth.com**

Lyles, Tennessee
Wings of Eagles Healthy Living, Inc.
Vicki Warren, BBEC
Website: **www.wehliving.org**

Baltimore, Maryland
Healthy Home Arts, LLC
Jennifer Michalack, BBEC
Website: **www.healthyhomearts.com**

Battle Creek, Michigan
Mike Weston
Email: **westonmf@comcast.net**

St. Paul, Minnesota
Damon Coyne
E-Mail:damon@intentionalenvironment.com
Website: **intentionalenvironment.com**

Other EMF/EMR Consultants

CANADA

South Western British Columbia
ElectroSmogSolutions
Chris Anderson & Associates,
EMR consultant following the Building Biology principles since 1999.
Website: **www.ElectroSmogSolutions.ca**

USA

Boulder, Colorado
Radsafe
Stan Hartman
Environmental health testing specializing in electro-magnetic fields and radiation.
Email: stan@radsafe.net
Website: **www.radsafe.net**

UK / NATIONWIDE

Offices in: Surrey, Yorkshire & Powys
Electric Forester Investigations Ltd.
Roger Moller BSc - Principal Investigator
On-Site and Remote Electromagnetic Surveys & Investigations
Homes, offices, factories and other built environments
Email: surveys@electricforester.co.uk
Website: **www.electricforester.co.uk**

EUROPE

Esslingen, Switzerland
Peter Schlegel
EMF/EMR testing of buildings; consulting in shielding; publicity & presentations in the field of EMF/EMR protection
Email: info@buergerwelle-schweiz.org
Website: **www.buergerwelle-schweiz.org**

AUSTRALIA

EMF/EMR Testing:

Tasmania/Melbourne:
EMFacts Consultancy
Don Maisch, PhD
Email: dmaisch@emfacts.com
Website: **www.emfacts.com**

Sydney:
EMR Surveys
John Lincoln
Email: emrsurveys@optusnet.com.au
Website: **www.emrsurveys.com.au**

Sydney:
EMR Australia
Lyn McLean
Email: contact@emraustralia.com.au
Website: **www.emrandhealth.com.au**

Melbourne, Victoria
Magshield Products, Intl.
Garry Melik
Email: **gmelik@magshield.com.au**

Melbourne, Victoria (Australia-wide)
Brookes EMS Pty Ltd.
Ken Brookes
Email: ken@brookes.com.au
Website: **www.brookesems.com.au**

Testing and Shielding Equipment

First, here is a brief description of each item; followed by sources listed by country.

Frequency Detection:

RF meters detect radio and microwave frequencies from mobile phones, wireless devices etc.

Electric Field meters detect lower frequencies from plugged-in devices, wiring etc.

Protective Shielding:

> **Air Tube, RF-Reducing Cell Phone** – The sound travels up the plastic air tube, limiting the amount of radiation to your brain from either cell phones or portable phones. If you must use a cell phone, using this headset will reduce radiation to the brain significantly.
>
> **Bed Canopies** – People who are electrically sensitive find shielding bed canopies essential, as do high performance athletes and, increasingly, business executives bathed in frequencies all day. Must be done properly; the material cannot rest on you and/or the bed.
>
> **Shielding Fabrics** – Shielding fabric by the foot can be used to line curtains, walls and can even be put under carpets or desk chair pads to shield from the wireless radiation of neighbors downstairs.
>
> **Shielding Films** – Placing plastic shielding film on glass windows can significantly block out ambient radio-frequency radiation-from where it comes into the building most easily.
>
> **Shielding Paints** – Metallic water-based paint can be placed under latex paints or wallpapers. Suitable for many types of exterior surfaces as well. Caution: The surface of this paint is highly conductive. It does need to be grounded and should <u>not</u> be installed without the services of an electrician.
>
> Also, do <u>not</u> put shielding paint on the walls if the room will contain RF emitting devices, such as computers, cell phones, wireless routers, compact fluorescent bulbs, etc.

CANADA

Safe Living Technologies
Website: **www.safelivingtechnologies.ca**

> **RF Meters:**
> RF Detector
> A broadband detector allows you to hear and assess all the invisible microwave emissions around you.

Electric Field Meters:
eME3030B Dual Function Gauss Meter/Tesla Meter and Electric Field Detector

Shielding Materials – A full line of bed canopies, fabrics, window foil and paint.

Air tube, RF-Reducing Cell Phone Headsets – Avoid the health hazards of traditional headsets. This headset allows for safer cell phone use.

Demand Switches – These products eliminate Electric and Magnetic fields in living spaces by automatically shutting off the power when it is not being used.

Shielded Power Cord – Help reduce electric fields by replacing your existing power cords with shielded power cords.

USA

EMF Safety Store
Website: **www.emfsafetystore.com**

RF & Other Meters:

ELECTROSMOG METER (RF Fields)
Very Sensitive, Affordable RF/MW Meter

ZAP CHECKER (RF Fields)
Economical, Fast, Extremely Sensitive RF/MW

4180 ELF GAUSS METER (Magnetic Fields)

BUDGET BUZZ STICK (Magnetic Fields)
This little unit won't actually measure anything numerically, but is a great sniffer-out of magnetic fields, letting you listen to them.

ELFLX DETECTOR (Electric Fields)

AC Electric Field Finder

This inexpensive little unit has no numerical readout, but will detect AC electric fields from 100 to 600 volts (50-60 Hz), displaying them with a red LED and an audio output.

Air tube RF-Reducing Cell Phone Headsets.

UK/EUROPE:

Sensory Perspective

Website: **www.detect-protect.com**

RF Meters

HF32D – Digital Microwave Analyser for 800-2500 MHz - For a quick and competent digital assessment of microwave exposure between 800 MHz and 2.5 GHz. This range includes mobile/cellular phones, cordless phones, Wi-MAX, Bluetooth, and computer/broadband wLANs.

Electric Field Meters

ELF-3030B - Digital ELF Meter for E & H Fields 16Hz-2kHz

Sensitive and informative, with digital display and sounder, it allows you to check electromagnetic radiation from the delivery and use of electricity around you.

Shielding Materials – a full line of bed canopies, fabrics, wallpaper and paint, clothing and demand switches.

Publications

The Powerwatch Handbook – Simple Ways to Make Your (EMF) Environment Safer (this is highly recommended.)

Please visit our website: www.radiationrescue.org for the following:

1. List of Recommended Books

2. Evidence of Harm – Reference Material, including these documents:

- *Summarizing the Science*– by Dr. Henry Lai. For those who argue there's not enough science to link electro-magnetic radiation exposure and health effects, here is a summary from one the most qualified scientists in this field. Dr. Lai details studies conducted over the past twenty years. Many of these show that EMR can affect cancers, immunology, genetics, cellular & molecular biology, behavior, reproduction and growth, hormones, the nervous system, the blood-brain barrier and metabolism.

- *Key Studies* cited by Dr. Sarah Starkey. This neuroscientist offers an extensive list of published studies detailing adverse health effects from EMR exposure. Dr. Starkey is a strong advocate of safer-tech solutions for schools and encourages them to replace harmful Wi-Fi networks with wired and/or fiber optics. Website: www.wifiinschools.org.uk

- *Cellphones and Brain Tumors – 15 Reasons for Concern*, August 2009, Primary Author: L. Lloyd Morgan, USA, Bioelectromagnetics Society, Electronics Engineer (retired) The full BioInitiative Report can be found at: www.bioinitiative.org/report index.htm

- *Symptoms of Electro-Magnetic Hypersensitivity – a Detailed List with References* From Larry Gust Environmental. This is a comprehensive document and very informative. Website: www.healbuildings.com

- *Breast Cancer Risks and EMR Exposure* – a list of published studies. This potential cause of breast cancer is not well known, but should be. (A woman should never carry a mobile phone in her bra, or anywhere on her body, when the mobile is in its sending/receiving mode.)

- *Scientists' Concerns About Wireless in Schools* An Open Letter to Parents, Teachers, School Boards. Regarding Wi-Fi Networks in Schools - May 5, 2009 by Dr. Magda Havas, Associate Professor, Trent University. Websites: www.magdahavas.com and www.doctorsforsaferschools.org

- *Wireless in the Air - Health and Safety Concerns* The full letter written to airline executives by Dr. Hans Scheiner and the German Environmental Physician Initiative. (When booking, please ask for Wi-Fi free flights.)

Index

Symbols

4-day Radiation Rescue 49
7 Key Reminders 221, 345

A

Abell, Robert (ND, LAc) 353
absorption of electro-magnetic radiation 55
Acid-Alkaline Diet 299
AC magnetic fields 60
ADD 38, 103, 243, 266, 272
Adey, Dr. Ross 32, 33, 70
ADHD 38, 103, 254, 263, 272, 274, 276, 277, 352, 353
ADSL modem/router 158
airplane travel 182–183, 209. *See also* aviation and EMR concerns
in-flight video screens 211
airport security scanners 182–183
alarm clocks/clock radios 199
Clocks - Safer Solutions 199
allergies 97, 167, 246, 247, 252, 265, 276, 299, 308
ALS 38, 39, 102, 246, 270, 276. *See also* neurological
Alzheimer's 10, 33, 38, 102, 254, 270, 281. *See also* neurological
American Academy of Anti-Aging Medicine (A4M) 293
American Environmental Health Foundation (AEHF) 244
Anderson, Chris 119, 159, 276
angina 35. *See also* cardiac symptoms, conditions and recommendations
anti-aging 39–40, 253, 293, 346
antioxidant nutritional supplements 177, 285
Arnetz, Dr. Bengt 262
arrhythmia 2, 35. *See also* cardiac symptoms, conditions and recommendations
Asperger's Syndrome 38, 223, 272
asthma 242, 247, 252, 253
Australasian College of Nutritional and Environmental Medicine 90
Australia 90, 350, 360
autism 4, 38, 39, 92, 102, 223, 254, 271, 272, 274, 275, 276, 277, 278, 279, 280, 281, 282, 283, 285, 298, 335, 352, 353
Autism Spectrum Disorders 38
autism resources 352
EMR, mercury and autism 280

NMT & Autism 298
aviation and EMR concerns 17, 107, 118, 182, 209–215, 365

B

baby monitors 194, 336
Baby Monitors - Safer Solutions 195
baby sensor pads/bedding 195
Baby Sensor Pads/Bedding - Safer Solutions 197
baby's room 193
Baerlocher, Mark (MD) 180
Balch, James (MD) 181
Balch, Phyllis A. (CNC) 181
Balmori, Alfonso (PhD) 74
Ban The Tower 90, 351
Bateman, Robert 317
Becker, Robert (MD) 6, 11, 175, 292, 327
bed canopies 218
Benetti, Dr. 40
bio-electrical field 92
BioInitiative Working Group/Report 77, 86, 87, 88, 249, 347
Biological Dentistry 287
Biological Dentists 357
biological effects 31, 45, 46, 53, 141, 365
birds' ability to migrate 72
birth defects 268
Bittar, Richard (MD) 90
Blackman, Dr. Carl 33
Blank, Martin (PhD) 10, 18, 31–32, 60, 61, 79, 82, 164, 237
blood-brain barrier 36, 45, 46, 53, 210, 243, 281, 285, 298, 365
Bluetooth®/bluetooth 68, 122, 127, 159, 207, 364. *See also* wireless headsets
Boham, Elizabeth (MD) 353
Boland, Andrea 82
BRAG™ Antenna Ranking 65
brain cancer 8, 22, 43–45, 47, 48, 50–51, 54, 58, 78, 100, 365
brain cells v, 6, 28, 40, 192, 281
breast cancer 40, 233, 264, 365

C

calming the scattered mind 304
Canada 88, 358, 359, 362
Canadian Initiative to Stop Wireless, Electric, and Electromagnetic Pollution (WEEP) 88, 247, 251, 349

Global Positioning Systems (GPS) 207
Goodman, Dr. Reba 31–32
Good Morning America 311
Gothenburg 90
grounding exercise 292
guidelines on RF exposures 77
Guinea Pigs "R" Us 88, 348
Gustavs, Katharina 17, 18, 64, 65, 119
Gust, Larry 18, 119, 123, 150, 194, 253, 278, 358, 365

H

H1N1 166
hair dryers 197
   Hair Dryers - Safer Solutions 199
Haley, Boyd (PhD) 280, 281, 285
Halmoy, Sissel (MS) 90
Hardell, Professor Lennart 29, 55, 100
Harkin, Senator Tom 81, 82
Hartman, Stan 18, 119, 122, 145, 203, 217, 218, 360
Haumann, Thomas (PhD) 46
Havas, Magda (PhD) 18, 28, 48, 65, 88, 165, 171, 242, 343, 347, 357, 365
headaches 38, 51, 97, 103, 159, 167, 171, 172, 187, 210, 223, 243, 247, 249, 290, 297, 300
headsets. *See* wireless headsets
Health Action Network (HANS) 348
Health Canada 54
heart. *See* cardiac symptoms, conditions and recommendations
heartburn and other stomach and digestive problems 300
Herberman, Dr. Ronald B. 47, 48, 137
Herouville-St.Clair 86
HESE (human ecological social economical project) 89, 350
high voltage power lines 15
Hoch, Christine 88, 348
hormones 33
hotel/motel accommodations 215
hot tubs 200
household appliances 192
Hughes, Carol (MP) 84
hybrid cars 204
   Hybrid Cars - Safer Solutions 205
Hydroxy L-tryptophan (5-HTP) 263
Hyman, Dr. Carrie (LAc, OMD) 18, 34, 137, 295, 344, 354
Hyman, Mark (MD) 254, 353
hypertension 2, 35

I

IARC: International Agency for Research on Cancer 78
IBE Certified Consultants 358
ICEMS: International Commission for Electromagnetic Safety 87, 351
IC-ESP: The International Coalition for an Electromagnetic Safe Planet 351
ICNIRP: International Commission on Non-Ionizing Radiation Protection 77
IEMFA: International EMF Alliance x, 88, 90, 351
immune system 32, 34, 58, 166, 214, 241, 242, 246, 251, 254, 255, 257, 262, 284, 287, 288, 296, 297, 308
Immune System Impairment 251
infertility 50, 256, 268
inflamed gums 300
in-flight video screens 211
insomnia 223, 243, 247, 249, 256, 257, 259, 260, 263, 265, 295, 300
Institute for Health and the Environment at the University of Albany 47
Internet access 122
   Safer Internet Access Solutions 158
   wireless Internet access 157
Internet Safety 312
Interphone Study 29
Ireland 349
Irish Doctors' Environmental Association (IDEA) 349
irritability 300
itching 300

J

Jabari, Talal 20
Johansson, Olle (PhD) 9, 18, 25, 39, 53, 57, 58, 100, 165, 182, 270, 332

K

Kabat-Zinn. Dr. Jon 304
Karlsson, Anne-Li 90
Karolinska Institute 262
Kartzinel, Dr. Jerry (MD) 281
Kelley, Elizabeth (MA) 87
Kelsey, Frances (MD) 76
Kenton, William 72
Key to the Safer Solutions 122
Khurana, Vini (MD) 19, 50, 66, 90
King, Larry 50–51
Klinghardt, Dietrich (MD) 19, 275, 276, 281, 284, 285, 299, 354
Kucinich, Congressman Dennis 82

Health Journey
Quality of Life
Killing You Softly